USMLE STEP 3 IN ONE WEEK

USMLE STEP 3 IN ONE WEEK

"USMLE" is a registered trademark of the National Board of Medical Examiners. The NBME is not affiliated with "USMLE Step 3 in one week".

NOTICE

Medicine is an ever-changing science. As new research expand our knowledge changes in treatment is necessary. The author has checked with sources and believes the information in this work is accurate however, human error or changes in medical science is possible. The author disclaim all responsibility for any errors or omissions or for the results obtained from use of the information contained in this work.

To the memory of my parents

To my wife my best companion and friend & to my children

USMLE STEP 3 IN ONE WEEK

Contents

Cardiology	8
Respiratory diseases	24
Rheumatology	32
Hematology	42
Gastrointestinal diseases	56
Neurology	74
Nephrology	86
Infectious & immune diseases	98
Endocrinology	114
Oncology	124
Dermatology	128

USMLE STEP 3 IN ONE WEEK

Surgery	**138**
Pediatrics	**156**
Obstetrics & gynecology	**186**
Psychiatry, ethics & intoxication	**218**

USMLE STEP 3 IN ONE WEEK

Cardiology

What is the significance of cardiac index?	Cardiac output with respect to body surface area (normal value 3-4)
Why do you have to follow up bicuspid valves?	Danger of aortic root dilatation causing aneurysm and dissection of aorta; 1st degree relatives needs echo
A diastolic murmur, plop sound, fever & thromboembolism what is the next step?	Echo to rule out myxoma
What is considered positive family history in coronary artery disease?	Male <55 Female <65
What is the management of bradycardia in inferior wall MI?	If asymptomatic wait for 24 hours since majority of them are self-limited. If symptomatic give atropine and if it didn't help use pacemaker
What is the next step if edema develops after CCB treatment for hypertension? Why?	You can add ACEI which acts on post capillary while CCB work on precapillary
What are the main differences in the management of STEMI vs. NSTEMI?	In NSTEMI only anticoagulation and in STEMI PCA or thrombolysis
What is the next step after a pt. arrives with chest pain?	If risk factors ,age, gender, clinical presentation and pretest probability suggest CAD treat the patient first
If ECG and CXR is negative in chest pain what is the next step?	Cardiac enzymes; rule out other causes of chest pain including pulmonary embolism and pericarditis
What is the best initial management for chest pain?	ECG, CXR and aspirin unless aortic dissection is suspected

USMLE STEP 3 IN ONE WEEK

What are the risk factors of CAD?	Diabetes, HTN, smoking, PAD, hyperlipidemia, obesity, positive family history, inactivity
What is the most common cause of non-cardiac chest pain apart from musculoskeletal causes?	GERD
What is the best initial test in CAD?	EKG unless the case is very typical for which aspirin is the first thing to do
What is the most accurate test in CAD?	Troponin every 6 hours & CK-MB
What are the differences between troponin and CK-MB?	Troponin 1-2 days, CK 1-2 weeks stay high
Which marker is increased first in CAD?	Myoglobin (1-4h)
What is the next step in the management of an atypical case of CAD and all tests are negative?	Stress testing
When do you order angiography in CAD suspected cases?	Only after stress test is abnormal
How do you perform stress test if the patient can't do on treadmill?	Adenosine, dobutamine, dipyridamole
How is the stress testing different in women?	Higher number of false positives in female patients
What are the cases that the patient can't go on the treadmill?	COPD, previous stroke, dementia, amputation, obesity, weakness, lower extremity ulcer
What are the indications of exercise thallium or stress echocardiography tests?	LBBB, digoxin, pacemaker, LVH, ST segment baseline abnormalities
When do you use sestamibi nuclear tests?	Obese patient with large breasts
What is more dangerous a	Reversible ischemia

USMLE STEP 3 IN ONE WEEK

fixed or reversible ischemia?	
What is the best test for ejection fraction?	MUGA (multigated acquisition scan)
What is the best test for valvular disease or wall motion?	Echo
What is acute coronary syndrome?	Acute chest pain suggesting STEMI, NSTEMI & unstable angina
What is the treatment of acute coronary syndrome?	MONA plus angioplasty or tPA (morphine, O2, nitrates and aspirin)
How is aspirin lowering mortality in acute coronary syndrome?	25% decrease mortality from acute MI and 50 decrease in mortality from unstable angina
What is the first medical contact to balloon time period?	Within 90 minutes of arrival or 120 minutes if the first medical facility was non PCI capable
What is the thrombolytic time frame?	Within 12h of pain & within 30 minutes of arrival
What conditions are needed to start thrombolytics?	ST elevation in 2 leads or new LBBB plus within 12h of pain
How do you manage STEMI?	NABAS Nitrates Aspirin and clopidogrel Beta blockers Anticoagulation Statins
What measures decrease mortality in acute coronary syndrome?	Aspirin, angioplasty, beta blockers, tPA, statins, clopidogrel
What are the contraindications of beta	Low blood pressure, bradycardia, overt CHF, severe COPD or asthma

blockers?	
Patient with stent needs to be warned about what serious consequences?	Stent thrombosis. They must receive aspirin and Prasugrel/clopidogrel and be warned of noncompliance
When do you give clopidogrel in CAD?	Angioplasty, aspirin allergy, in combination with aspirin for unstable angina, post stent
When Ca channel blockers are indicated in CAD?	If beta blockers are contraindicated (e.g. asthma), cocaine use, Prinzmetal angina
What medication is contraindicated if cocaine induced chest pain is suspected?	Beta blockers worsen the situation by unopposed effect of alpha causing more vasoconstriction
If cocaine induced chest pain is suspected and no ECG abnormalities are seen, what is the next step?	Benzodiazapines and if they don't help alpha blockers such as phentolamine
When is pacemaker indicated?	3rd degree block, Mobitz type II, symptomatic bradycardia, new LBBB, bifascicular block
Why do we see hypotension post MI?	Arrhythmia (3rd degree block or sinus bradycardia), shock, rupture (valve, septum, wall), RV infarction
What are the diagnostic tests and management of cardiogenic shock?	Echo, Swan-Ganz, ACE inhibitors, urgent revascularization
What is the management of valve rupture?	Echo, ACEI, nitroprusside, intraaortic balloon counterpulsation as a bridge to surgery
How do you manage septal rupture?	Echo, Catheterization, ACE inhibitors, nitroprusside, surgery
What specific adverse effect of sodium Nitroprusside is of note?	Cyanide toxicity
How do you manage wall	Echo, tap pericardium, urgent surgery

rupture?

What is the management of sinus bradycardia?	EKG, atropine and if necessary pacemaker
How do you diagnose and manage 3rd degree block?	EKG, Cannon a wave seen on JVP, atropine and pacemaker if needed
What is the management for right ventricle MI?	Check BP regularly and if low give fluids, don't use nitrates, the rest of treatment is the same as other types of MI
What prescription is given to a post-MI discharge?	Aspirin and/or clopidogrel, beta blockers, ACE inhibitors and statins
When do you stop statins if myopathy develops?	Only if CK is more than 10 times the normal value otherwise recheck CK value after a week
When can the patient with MI resume sexual activity?	If there is no pain following mild activities can resume sex in 3 weeks
How do you manage NSTEMI?	No need for thrombolytics, heparin, GP IIb/IIIa inhibitors especially if angioplasty is needed
When do GP IIb/IIIa inhibitors have most benefits?	With angioplasty
What are the side effects of ACE inhibitors/ ARBs?	Both cause hyperkalemia, only ACE inhibitors cause cough
How do you treat stable angina?	Aspirin, beta blockers, nitrates if pain, ACE inhibitors if EF is low, CHF or systolic dysfunction
Why do we do angiography?	To select CABG candidates and do angioplasty when appropriate
What are the indications for CABG?	Left main, triple vessel disease (>70% occlusion) esp. when proximal ADA is involved, refractory angina
What differentials should be considered in sudden	CAD, valvular dis., HOCM, arrhythmia, Long QT, WPW, Brugada, and Anomaly of origin

cardiac death?	of coronary arteries (from venous blood)
What is Brugada syndrome?	ST elevation in V1-V3 and incomplete RBBB, also syncope, fever and A. Fib can be seen
What are the CAD equivalents?	Diabetes, PAD, carotid disease, aortic disease
What risk of atherosclerotic cardiovascular disease (ASCVD) is needed for statin therapy?	7.5 % or higher
What is the difference between high and moderated intensity statin treatment?	High intensity is either atorvastatin 40-80 or rosuvastatin 20-40 mg. Medium intensity is ¼ dose of high intensity
Who needs statins if they have diabetes?	Everybody between 40-75 years of age
What LDL level is treated in every patient?	190; also any pt. with significant arterioscleriotic events regardless of LDL level
What are the 5 risk factors for hyperlipidemia?	HTN, smoking, Low HDL, age and family history
What age is a risk factor for hyperlipidemia?	Male >45, female >55
How low should HDL be to be considered a risk factor for hyperlipidemia?	<40
What level of triglycerides does need treatment?	- Above 1000 needs fibrates and if they can't tolerate that fish oil or niacin - 150-500 don't need therapy if no ASCVD is present however, if they are taking statins for other causes it can help with triglyceride levels

USMLE STEP 3 IN ONE WEEK

	also
What is the best method to diagnose CHF?	Clinical diagnosis: 2 major or 1 major and 2 minor Framingham criteria
What are the major criteria for CHF?	PND, JVP, Rales, S3, pulmonary edema, cardiomegaly Hepatojugular reflux Weight loss >4.5 kg in 5 days in response to treatment
What are the minor criteria for CHF?	b/l ankle edema, pleural effusion, hepatomegaly, exertional SOB, nocturnal cough, HR>120, low vital capacity
What is the treatment of acute pulmonary edema?	MOND: morphine, O2, nitrates, diuretics (furosemide)
What is the significance of BNP?	Negative test rules out CHF
At what age do we need to check cholesterol level in every patient?	Everybody at 20 needs to check cholesterol level and after that every 5 years. If one parent has high cholesterol check at very early age
How do you calculate LDL?	Total cholesterol – HDL – VLDL (TG/5)
What diagnostic tests do you use for CHF?	CXR (cardiomegaly, effusion, pulmonary congestion and cephalization), EKG, Echo, pulse oximetry (hypoxia, respiratory alkalosis), consider ABG after pulse oximetry
Where do you admit MI and pulmonary edema?	ICU
Pulmonary edema not improving 30 min. after MOND therapy (morphine, O2, Nitrates, diuretics) What's the next step?	Positive inotropics (dobutamine, milrinone
When do you use unsynchronized	Ventricular fibrillation, Ventricular tachycardia with no pulse

cardioversion?	
What is nesiritide?	Atrial natriuretic factor (synthetic) used in acute pulmonary edema
What are the 2 beta blockers that decrease mortality in CHF?	Metoprolol and carvedilol
When does spironolactone decrease mortality in CHF?	Only is class III and IV heart failure
How do you treat CHF with diastolic dysfunction?	Beta blockers and diuretics
How do you treat acute CHF with pulmonary edema?	NNN: nitroglycerin, Nitroprusside and nesiritide
What is the management of heart failure?	ACEI/ARB, diuretics, beta blockers, and if EF<30% spironolactone and ICD Digoxin is given if spironolactone can't help with symptoms
What medications increase digoxin toxicity?	VAQS: verapamil, amiodarone, quinidine and spironolactone
What reduces mortality in CHF?	ABS: ACE inhibitors, beta blockers, spironolactone
When does ICD indicated in CHF?	When EF is less than 35 % implantable cardioverter defibrillator is indicated
What are the indications of ICD?	Family history of sudden cardiac death, sustained spontaneous ventricular arrhythmia, recurrent syncope or syncope with exercise, HOCM, CHF(low EF)
What is the most common cause of death in CHF?	Arrhythmia causing sudden death
When do you use biventricular pacemaker?	When ORS > 130 ms
Is there any indication for warfarin in heart failure?	None
What is the absolute contraindication for beta blockers?	Symptomatic bradycardia
What percentage of	60 %

asthmatics does tolerate beta blockers well?	
What increases all murmurs of the right heart?	Inhalation
What increases all murmurs of the left heart?	Exhalation
What are the two murmurs that are decreased by squatting and leg raise?	HOCM, MVP
What are the functions of amyl nitrates in evaluating murmurs?	Decreases afterload (like ACE inhibitors); it increases aortic stenosis murmur by increasing flow through the stenotic valve
What is the function of handgrip in evaluating murmurs?	Increases afterload
What murmurs gets louder with Valsalva maneuver?	HOCM and MVP murmurs are increased
What valve diseases need ACE inhibitors?	Any aortic or mitral regurgitation and VSD
What is the most common presentation for aortic stenosis?	Chest pain
What is the size of aortic valve orifice in severe aortic stenosis?	<1 Cm
What signs are seen in severe aortic stenosis?	Load and Late murmur, late pulse
What is the survival rate for aortic stenosis?	If coronary ischemia is present 3-5, syncope 2-3 years, CHF 1.5-2 years
What is the normal aortic valve gradient?	<30 is normal, 30-70 is moderate and >70 is severe stenosis
How do you treat aortic stenosis?	Initial treatment is diuretics but they need surgery

What INR is used for mechanical aortic valve?	2-3 except for the first 3 months after surgery or if there is risk factors for thromboembolisms which require 2.5-3.5
What INR is used for mechanical mitral valve?	2.5-3.5 (remember **M**itral needs **M**ore)
What are the causes of aortic regurgitation?	HTN, rheumatic fever, infective endocarditis, cystic medical necrosis, Marfan's, Reiter's, syphilis, ankylosing spondylitis
What are the classical findings in aortic regurgitation?	Quincke pulse (nail), Corrigan pulse (water hammer), Musset's sign (head moving by each pulse), Duroziez's sign (femoral murmur), Hill sign (lower extremity gradient increases)
What is the most common presentation of aortic regurgitation?	Fatigue and shortness of breath
How do you compare the accuracy of echocardiography and cardiac catheterization?	Transthoracic (TTE) < transesophageal (TEE) < cardiac catheterization
What are the causes of mitral regurgitation?	Acute MI, trauma, anything that causes dilation of the heart, rheumatic fever, infective endocarditis, MVP
What characteristics do mitral regurgitation murmurs have?	They obscure S1 and S2
How do you treat mitral regurgitation?	Diuretics, ACE inhibitors, nifedipine, surgery if **EF<60%** or LV end systolic diameter is >45 mm
In what age group S3 is normal?	<30
What is the significance of almost normal EF in mitral regurgitation?	Not a good sign and surgery needed since mitral regurgitation is associated with high EF
What is the treatment of ASD?	If shunt ratio is > 1-1.5 percutaneous method or catheter device is used
What is Kussmaul's sign?	JVP is increased on inspiration

USMLE STEP 3 IN ONE WEEK

What is the next step in a patient with dilated cardiac chamber on echo? Rule out ischemic cause of dilated cardiomyopathy by doing stress test

What are the diagnostic hallmarks of restrictive cardiomyopathy? Low voltage EKG, catheterization (rapid x and y descents)

What is the treatment of restrictive cardiomyopathy? Diuretics

What EKG changes are pathognomonic for pericarditis? PR segment depression

How do you treat pericarditis? NSAIDs initially and if they don't get better in 24-48h use prednisone

EKG shows low voltage with electrical alternans and all pressures on cardiac catheterization are equal, what is the diagnosis? Temponade

What is the most dangerous therapy for temponade? Diuretics

What are the differentials for Kussmaul's sign? Constrictive pericarditis and restrictive CMP

When do you see low voltage EKG? Restrictive CMP, cardiac temponade, constrictive pericarditis

How do you diagnose constrictive pericarditis? High JVP, prominent y descent, ascites, edema, CXR (calcification), EKG (low voltage), CT/MRI shows thickening

What is the treatment for constrictive pericarditis? Diuretics and surgery

What is the diagnosis when there is pressure difference between right and left arm? Dissecting aortic aneurysm

What is the best initial test CXR however the most accurate test is CT

USMLE STEP 3 IN ONE WEEK

for dissecting aortic aneurysm?	angiography. You can use TEE or MRI too
What size of aorta is needed for diagnosing AAA?	3 Cm
Is there any screening test for abdominal aortic aneurysm?	Male 65 >who has ever smoked need ultrasonography
What is the best initial test for peripheral artery disease?	Ankle/brachial index 0.9 or less
What is the most accurate test for PAD?	Angiography
How do you treat PAD?	Aspirin, exercise as tolerated, statins, BP control and screening for diabetes. Cilostazol is used if exercise didn't help, if not improving surgery
How do you manage acute limb ischemia?	If negative pulse on Doppler and severe pain with delayed capillary refill emergency revascularization needed otherwise after 6 hours tissue dies
What is the mechanism of action of cilostazol?	Blocks PDE3 which increases cAMP and protein kinase which leads to inhibition of platelet aggregation
When do you operate on carotid stenosis?	- Symptomatic and 50% stenosis - Asymptomatic: 60% in male and 70% in female
What diagnosis must be rule out if there is unilateral Horner's and sudden headache?	Carotid artery dissection
What tests do you need to order for atrial fibrillation?	TSH, T4, electrolytes, CK-MB and troponin, Echo, EKG, telemetry, Holter's monitoring
When do we call the patient hemodynamically unstable?	Hypotension, confusion, chest pain, CHF

USMLE STEP 3 IN ONE WEEK

How do you treat atrial fibrillation?	- Rate control - rhythm conversion - anticoagulation
How do you determine if anticoagulation is needed for atrial fibrillation?	if CHADS score is 2 or more as long as it persists more than 2 days (INR 2-3 is desired)
What medications are used for rate control in atrial fibrillation?	BCD: beta blockers, CCB, digoxin
How do you convert the A. fib rhythm?	cardioversion if it is new onset and acute; amiodarone
What is CHADS-VAS?	CHF, Hypertension, Age 75 and more, DM, Stroke, Vascular diseases, Age 65-74, female sex Every risk factor gets 1 point except for age 75 and stroke which get 2 points CHADS are 0: no anticoagulation CHADS is 2: oral anticoag. CHADS is 1: aspirin or oral anticoagulation or do nothing
What is the treatment for atrial flutter?	BCD: beta blocker if IHD, migraine, Grave's disease or pheochromocytoma present; calcium channel blockers for asthma or migraine; digoxin for borderline hypotension
What is multifocal atrial tachycardia?	3 or more polymorphic P waves, MCC is hypoxia & COPD Low Mg, low K, CAD, HTN, valvular dis. can cause that too Rate is >100 Treat the underlying disease however, verapamil can help
What is SVT (supraventricular tachycardia?	Rate is 160-180 if regular rhythm
How do you treat SVT?	If stable use vagal maneuvers, adenosine and cardiac ablation for persistent cases; if unstable shock
What is WPW?	Wolf Parkinson White is SVT that alternates

	with V. tach, shows delta wave, gets worse with CCB or digoxin, most accurate test is electrophysiology studies
What is the significance of atrial fibrillation and WPW?	Very dangerous since every atrial impulse is going to the ventricles without AV node delay
How do you treat WPW?	Vagal maneuvers, Procainamide, cardioversion, ablation
How do you treat table V. tach?	Amiodarone / lidocaine/ procainamide/ Mg
What is the treatment for Torsade?	Mg sulfate and if no response temporary pacing
What are the causes of long QT syndrome?	Medications, ischemic heart disease, HIV, intracranial diseases, bradyarrhythmia, hypothermia, starvation, hypothyroidism
What medications do cause long QT?	Antipsychotics (esp. quetiapine), TCA, SSRI, antiarrhythmic (sotalol, amiodarone, flacainide), antibiotics
How do you treat V. fibrillation?	Start with PCR and shock then drugs (amiodarone or lidocaine) then shock and drugs is repeated and finally shock the patient for the 3rd time, between shocking the patient continue with PCR
How do you evaluate syncope?	Gradual vs. sudden loss of consciousness
What are the causes of sudden loss of consciousness?	cardiac vs. neurological ; if regains consciousness quickly it is arrhythmia otherwise structural causes like
What are the cardiac causes of syncope?	Structural vs. arrhythmia (regains consciousness quickly)
What are the structural cardiac causes of syncope?	Aortic stenosis, HOCM, MVP, mitral stenosis, MI and myxoma

How do you differentiate vasovagal syncope?	Usually associated with emotional, painful events or prolonged standing
What are the causes of gradual loss of consciousness?	toxic metabolic, hypoxia, hyperglycemia, anemia, drugs
What is the management of syncope?	Holter, telemetry, repeat troponin every 4-6 hours, urine toxicology, blood toxicology, tilt test and electrophysiology studies
How do you manage the patient if atrial fibrillation is the cause of syncope?	ICD
What etiology has the worst prognosis in syncope?	Cardiac origin
What beta blocker is used in the management of aortic dissection?	Esmolol since it has a very short half life

USMLE STEP 3 IN ONE WEEK

Respiratory Diseases

How do you diagnose asthma?	Symptomatic by spirometry(12 % improvement of FEV1 with bronchodilators) and asymptomatic by metacholine challenge test
What is mild asthma?	FEV1 or PEF 40% or more
What are the orders for shortness of breath?	O2, oximetry, CXR, ABG
How do you treat asthma?	Mild asthma SABA such as albuterol plus O2 is used first and if no response PO steroids; Moderate to severe: Methyl prednisolone, Albuterol, O2 and Ipratropium (MAOI) If respiratory arrest is about to happen add MgSO4, epinephrine and intubate
Which asthmatics go to ICU?	Asthmatics with CO2 retention
Which drugs have no clear benefit in the treatment of *acute* asthma?	Theophyllines, cromolyns, montelukast, omalizumab, long acting beta2 agonists
How do you treat non-acute forms of asthma?	First Inhaled beta agonist, then add inhaled corticosteroids, add long acting beta2 agonists and finally oral steroids
What is the main medication for hay fever?	Cromolyns
What medication does help atopy?	Montelukast

USMLE STEP 3 IN ONE WEEK

What medication acts against IgE?	omalizumab
What is the treatment of acute COPD?	MAOI(methylprednisolone, albuterol, O2, ipratropium) and antibiotics if fever and sputum exists(ceftriaxone plus azithromycin)
What is the next step in the treatment of acute COPD and mild acidosis if CO2 is still high, would you intubate?	No. Use CPAP OR BiPAP
What are the two main measures that decrease mortality in COPD?	Smoking cessation and long term O2 therapy
What is the treatment of exercise induced asthma?	Inhaled corticosteroids and montelukast?
How would you rate an asthmatic with Pco2 and Po2 of 50 and 50?	Moderate or severe asthma
Why do we see increase in DLCO in COPD?	Destruction of interstitium
When do we give home O2 therapy in COPD?	PO2<55 or O2 sat.<88
What is the treatment of alpha 1 AT deficiency?	Infusion of alpha 1 AT
What is the diagnois of emphysema in <40 years old plus increased INR & low albumin?	Alpha 1 AT deficiency
When do you intubate in COPD?	When acidosis gets worse

USMLE STEP 3 IN ONE WEEK

What is the most accurate test for bronchiectasis diagnosis?	High resolution CT
What is characteristic for bronchiectasis on CXR?	Tram tracking
How do you treat bronchiectasis?	Physiotherapy and rotating antibiotics
What commonly used antibiotic can cause interstitial lung disease?	Trimethoprim and sulfamethoxazole
What is the Byssinosis?	Interstitial lung disease caused by cotton
What is the diagnosis of Interstitial lung disease in electricians, ceramic workers, fluorescent bulb workers?	Berylliosis
Which interstitial lung disease is treatable?	Berylliosis
What is the implication of fever or systemic signs in suspected ILD?	ILD is ruled out
What pattern of spirometry is seen in ILD?	Everything is decreased except FEV1/FVC
What is the most common cancer in asbestosis?	Not mesothelioma, however asbestos is the most common cause of mesothelioma
What is the treatment of ILD?	Trial of steroids but only Berylliosis responds
What is the diagnosis of ILD pattern plus fever, constitutional symptoms and a fast course?	BOOP/COP (bronchiolitis obliterans organizing pneumonia)
How do you treat BOOP/COP?	Steroids(good response)
What is definitive diagnosis of BOOP/COP?	Open biopsy but CT and CXR helps
What is significance of ACE increase in serum?	Sarcoidosis
What are the diagnostic	Hypercalcemia, increase T helper cells in

clues in sarcoidosis?	bronchoalveolar lavage and ACE level
What is the best initial test in sarcoidosis?	CXR but most accurate is biopsy
What is the treatment of sarcoidosis?	Steroids if necessary
What is the most accurate test for pulmonary hypertension?	Cardiac catheterization, But echo and EKG helps
What are the treatment options for pulmonary hypertension?	Sildenafil, Calcium channel blockers(nifedipine), Epoprostenol, Bosentan(endothelin inhibitor)
What are the risk factors for pulmonary embolism?	MISTT: Malignancy, Immobilization, Surgery, Trauma and Thrombocytopenia
What is the significance of Well's criteria?	If more than 4 then pulmonary embolism is likely which necessitates spiral CT otherwise a low D-dimer rules out PE
What is Well's criteria?	- Cancer / hemoptysis 1 point each - Hx of DVT or PE / tachycardia /recent surgery or immobilization 1.5 points each - clinical DVT/no other Dx is likely 3 points each
How long is the duration of anticoagulation after DVT?	6 months if idiopathic 3-6 months if there is a risk factor
What is the differential diagnosis of thrombophilia?	Factor V Leiden, Protein C or S mutation, lupus anticoagulant
What is the most diagnostic EKG pattern for pulmonary embolism?	S in lead I, Q and T in lead III, however is seen occasionally
What are the common EKG patterns seen in pulmonary embolism?	Tachycardia, nonspecific ST and T changes, RBBB and right axis deviation
What CXR findings are seen in pulmonary embolism?	Atelectasis(common), wedge shaped infarct(rare)
What ABG results are	A-a gradient increase and alkalosis

seen in pulmonary embolism?	
If Doppler of the legs shows DVT do you do spiral CT as your next step?	No, start the patient on LMWH and treat as pulmonary embolism
What percentage of people with "high probability" V/Q scan result don't have pulmonary embolism?	15%
What is initial management for suspected pulmonary embolism?	Heparin, D-dimer, Doppler of legs and CXR. If CXR is positive or if Well's criteria is 4 or higher spiral CT
What is the most accurate test for pulmonary embolism?	Angiography but 0.5% mortality rate
When do you use IVC filter?	Contraindication to anticoagulation, thrombosis despite anticoagulation
How do you treat pulomanry embolisms?	O2, heparin, warfarin. If hemodynamically unstable fibrinolysis is given and if contraindication to anticoagulation is present IVC filter
What are the main elements of exudative pleural fluid analysis?	LDH>0.6 of serum level, Protein>0.5 of serum level
How do we treat pleural effusion?	If small amount no treatment or we can give diuretics. Chest tube, pleurodesis (bleomycin or talcum powder) and decortication
Pt. with daytime sleepiness, HTN, headache & erectile dysfunction?	Obstructive sleep apnea
How do you diagnose sleep apnea?	Polysomnography: 5-20 episodes of apnea is mild, 20-30 is moderate and more than 30 is severe

What is the treatment of sleep apnea?	Weight loss, CPAP/BiPAP and finally surgery
What is the treatment of central sleep apnea?	Avoid alcohol & sedatives, acetazolamide causes metabolic acidosis & stimulates respiratory center, medroxyprogesterone
A patient with respiratory symtoms ahs brownish mucus plug sputum, high eosinophils and IgE with central bronchiectasis, what is the diagnosis?	Allergic bronchopulmonary aspergillosis
How do you diagnose allergic bronchopulmonary aspergillosis?	Skin test, IgE test, Aspergillus fumigatus serology
What is the treatment of allergic bronchopulmonary aspergillosis?	Steroids; if refractory add itraconazole
What are the causes of ARDS?	Shock, trauma, pancreatitis, burns, aspiration, sepsis, near drowning and toxic inhalation
What is the treatment of ARDS?	PEEP with low tidal volume, Prone position, diuretics unless shock is the cause, ICU transfer and dobutamine
How do you diagnose ARDS?	CXR shows patchy infiltration, PO2/FIO2<200 and normal Swan Ganz wedge pressure
What Swan Ganz readings do you see in cardiogenic shock?	Cardiac output is low, wedge pressure is high, SVR is high
What is the most common cause of hospital acquired pneumonia?	Gram negative bacteria
What is the strongest indication of admission for pneumonia?	Respiratory distress

USMLE STEP 3 IN ONE WEEK

What is the pneumonia severity index?	Old age hypoxia must be admitted with or without fever. If severe hypoxia admit to ICU
When do you admit pneumonia to ICU?	Severe hypoxia
What orders do you write for pneumonia?	Oximetry, CXR, O2 if shortness of breath, ABG if hypoxia
What is the treatment of pneumonia?	Outpatient use quinolones or macrolides, inpatient azithromycin plus ceftriaxone
What is the treatment for ventilator associated pneumonia?	Vancomycin plus Zosyn(piperacillin plus tazobactam)
When do you give steroids in Pneumocystis pneumonia?	PO2<70 or A-a gradient >35
What disease is caused by Coxiella burneti?	Q fever, important to look for animal contact
When is a person with TB non-infectious?	If 3 sputums are negative
How do you treat TB?	RIPE(rifampin 6 months, Isoniazid 6 months, pyrazinamide 2 months, ethambutol 2 months
When do you treat TB for more than 6 months?	MMCOP: meningitis, miliary TB, cavitary TB, osteomyelitis and pregnancy
What do you do if PPD is positive even if there is history of TB vaccination?	9
What are 2 stages testing for TB?	If never tested or tested long time ago you test and if it is negative you repeat it after 1-

	2 weeks
How do you interpret PPD results?	5 mm is positive if close contact or immune deficient or CXR positive 10 mm is positive if high risk 15 mm is positive for every one
What is quantiferon test?	Measuring gamma interferon released by WBC after contact with TB Ag
What is the management of solitary lung nodule (coin lesion)?	If the pt. is high risk excision is the treatment. If low risk repeat CT. if intermediate risk and the size is at least 0.8 PET otherwise repeat CT.
What are the characteristics of a malignant pulmonary nodule?	Eccentric or reticular calcification Benign calcification is popcorn, laminated, diffuse or central calcifications
What is the screening test for lung cancer?	55-80 years old with 30 pack year smoker or quit less than 15 years ago, low dose CT yearly

Rheumatology

What are the common features of Ehlers Donlos syndrome and Marfan's?	Joint hypermobility, chest and spine deformities, MVP, AD inheritance (however, skin changes are seen in EDS while problems with lens, aortic valve and spontaneous pneumothorax are seen in Marfan's)
What is the significance of anti-CCP?	**Citrullinated cyclic peptide is very specific for rheumatoid arthritis**
What is Felty's syndrome?	Splenomegaly + rheumatoid arthritis
In what disease you see the lowest level of glucose?	Rheumatoid arthritis
Which joints are spared in rheumatoid arthritis?	Sacroiliac joints
How do you treat rheumatoid arthritis?	NSAIDS and DMARDS and maybe a short course of steroids if you want to subside the acute flare faster
What are the DMARDS?	Methotrexate, hydroxyl chloroquine, sulfasalazine, biological agents(anti TNF), gold, leflunomide, abetacept, anakirna
What are differentials of seronegative arthritis?	Seronegative(RF negative) diseases are: ankylosing spondylitis, psoriasis, reactive arthritis, juvenile rheumatoid arthritis
What are the complications	Uveitis and aortitis

of ankylosing spondylitis?

How do you diagnose ankylosing spondylitis?	MRI
What is the treatment of ankylosing spondylitis?	NSAIDS, sulfasalazine and biologic agents
What is reactive arthritis or Reiter's syndrome?	Arthritis, uveitis, urethritis or cervicitis, keratoderma balarrhagicum, circinate balanitis
What infections cause reactive arthritis?	CCYSS: Chlamydia, Campylobacter, Yersinia, Shigella, Salmonella
How do you treat Reiters?	NSAIDS
DIP joint involvement, sausage shaped fingers and nail pitting is seen in what disease?	Psoriasis
How do you treat psoriasis arthritis?	NSAIDS, Infliximab, methotrexate
What are the main features of JRA?	Fever, leukocytosis, hepatosplenomegaly, myalgia, transaminitis, increase ferritin, salmon colored rash, seronegative and negative ANA
How do you treat JRA?	NSAIDS, methotrexate
What is Whipple's disease?	Fever, malabsorption, BBBB(bacteria, bowel biopsy and Bactrim for treatment)
DIP nodes are characteristically seen in what disease?	Osteoarthritis

USMLE STEP 3 IN ONE WEEK

What are the main features of synovial fluid analysis in osteoarthritis?	Cell<2000 (in RA it is between 5 to 50 thousands
How do you treat osteoarthritis?	NSAIDS and glucosamine sulfate
What is the work up for SLE?	ANA(best initial test), Anti DS DNA & Anti Smith are the most specific
What is the best test for determining severity of SLE?	Decrease in complement and increase in anti-double stranded DNA
Anti- Smith Abs are seen in what disease?	SLE
What is the risk of having anti SS-A(Ro)?	Heart block
How do you treat SLE?	NSAID for joint pain, steroids for flare ups, antimalarial for rash and joint pain, mycophenolate for lupus nephritis, if after stopping steroids there is relapse use azathioprine and cyclophosphamide
What medications do cause drug induced lupus?	Hydralazine, INH , procainamide,
What are the main differences between SLE and drug induced lupus?	No renal or CNS involvement, presence of anti- histone Abs
What major cardiovascular concern is seen in SLE?	Very high risk of coronary artery disease
What disease causes loss of teeth and taste plus sicca syndrome?	Sjogren
How do you make the diagnosis of Sjogren?	Lip biopsy is the most accurate test, ANA is 95% sensitive, SSA(Ro) and SSB(La) are

	fairly specific
What lab tests are positive in ANA negative SLE?	SSA, SSB can be positive
How do you treat Sjogren?	M3 agonists like pilocarpine, cevimeline and use of moisturizing drops for the eyes and mouth
What malignancy is associated with Sjogren?	B cell lymphoma
What is the diagnosis of a patient with pruritus, dysphagia, joint involvement, malignant hypertension, pulmonary hypertension?	Systemic sclerosis
What lab tests are diagnostic for systemic sclerosis?	Both ANA(90%) and Scl-70(70%) are non-diagnostic.
What is the mechanism of bacterial overgrowth in systemic sclerosis?	Motility disorder
What percentage of CREST syndrome does show Scl-70?	None
How do you treat systemic sclerosis?	There is no effective treatment. ACEI for renal problems and pulmonary hypertension is treated with SCEB: Sildenafil, Calcium channel blockers(nifedipine), Epoprostenol, Bosentan(endothelin inhibitor)
What is CREST syndrome?	Calcinosis, Reynaud's, esophageal dismotility, sclerodactyly and telangiectasia
What organs are not	Heart, kidney, lung and joints

involved in CREST?

What is eosinophilic fasciitis? Orange peel skin, marked eosinophilia, no lung, heart and kidney involvement.

How do you treat eosinophilic fasciitis? Steroids

What is the difference between dermatomyositis and polymyositis? Skin involvement plus polymyosisit is dermatomyositis

How do you diagnose polymyositis? CK, aldolase and anti-Jo-1 helps but definite diagnosis is biopsy

What are the skin manifestations of dermatomyositis? Gottron's papules, Shawl sign and heliotrope rash around the eyes

What is the differential diagnosis for high aldolase? Muscle and liver injury

How do you diagnose fibromyalgia? Dx of exclusion
≥ 3 mo widespread b/l pain/tenderness above and below the waist & axial spine
Stiffness, fatigue; sleep problems, anxiety

What is the significance of anti-Jo-1? Increase chance of ILD

What is the most common complication of dermatomyositis? Malignancy

What is the treatment of dermatomyositis and polymyositis? Steroids

What is the treatment of fibromyalgia? Exercise, tricyclic antidepressants, gabapentin

How is the relationship between pain and weakness in polymyalgia rheumatica?	Pain is more prominent than weakness
What are the main features of polymyalgia rheumatica?	Over 50, female, proximal pain, high ESR, normal CK and aldolase, negative biopsy and amazing response to steroids
What are the differential diagnoses for polymyalgia rheumatic?	Fibromyalgia and chronic fatigue syndrome
What main change in platelet numbers is seen in vasculitides?	thrombocytosis
How do you treat vasculitis?	SCAM(steroids, cyclophosphamide, azathioprine, mecaptopurine and methotrexate)
What are the main features of polyarthritis nodosa?	PARTH(pericardium, abdomen, renal, testes involvement and hypertension) but no lung involvement
Best initial test for polyarthritis nodosa?	Abdominal angiography
What is the most accurate test for diagnosing PAN?	Biopsy of skin, muscle or sural nerve
How do you treat PAN and Wegener's?	Prednisone and cyclophosphamide
What is the relationship between PAN and HBsAg?	30% seen together
What test is diagnostic for Wegener's?	C-ANCA

USMLE STEP 3 IN ONE WEEK

Which disease does show p-ANCA?	Churge-Strauss
How do you treat Churg-Strauss disease?	Steroids
What is the differential for mononeuritis multiplex?	Diabetes, connective tissue diseases, vasculitis, Lyme, HIV, amyloid, cryoglobulinemia, drugs(dapsone)
What disease is seen in Asian female with diminished radial pulse?	Takayasau's
How do you diagnose Takayasau's?	Aortography or MRA(no need for biopsy)
What is the treatment of Takayasau's?	Steroids
What liver disease is associated with cryoglobulinemia?	Hepatitis C (treat with interferon alpha and ribavirin)
How do you treat Behcet's?	Prednisone and colchicine
What type of crystal is seen in Gouts?	Negative birefringence needle
What type of crystal is seen in pseudogouts?	Positive birefringence rhomboids
What is the most accurate test for gout pseudogouts and septic arthritis?	Aspiration : <2000 is normal; 2000-50000 is inflammatory like gout or pseudogout; >50000 is septic
What are the risk factors for gout exacerbation?	Beer binge, thiazides and nicotinic acid

What is characteristic for gout on toe X-ray?	Punched out lesions
Is uric acid level a reliable test in acute gouty arthritis?	No. 30% have normal UA level during attack which is the result of precipitation of UA and decrease UA level.
Is high uric acid level an indication of treating gouty arthritis?	No. Treatment isn't necessary if asymptomatic
How do you treat gout?	NSAIDS, steroids, colchicine(given if contraindication to NSAIDS) Intraarticular steroid injection in acute gout with chronic renal diseases
Can you use colchicine for gout prophylaxis?	Yes but side effects are limiting factors(GI upset and BM suppression)
How do you prevent gouty attacks?	Weights loss, avoid alcohol, allopurinol, probenecid, sulfinpyrazone and colchicine
What are the side effects of allopurinol?	Rash, interstitial nephritis, hemolysis
What are the predisposing factors for pseudogout?	HHHA: hypothyroidism, hemochromatosis, hyperparathyroidism and acromegaly
What are the most common sites for pseudogout?	Knee and wrist
What are the most common causes of septic arthritis?	Staph. aureus (40%), Strep. pyogens(30%), Gram negatives (20%)
What are the risk factors for septic arthritis?	Prosthetic joint, osteoarthritis, rheumatoid arthritis

USMLE STEP 3 IN ONE WEEK

How do you treat septic arthritis?	Vancomycin(G+) plus ceftriaxone(G-)
What is the hallmark of Paget's disease of bone?	Increased bone turnover: alkaline phosphatase and urinary hydroxyproline increases
What is the best initial test for Paget's?	Alkaline phosphatase
What is the most accurate test for Paget's?	X-ray shows lytic and blastic lesions
What are the calcium and phosphorus level in Paget's?	Normal calcium and phosphorus
How do you treat Paget's?	Bisphosphonates and calcitonin
What is the most important differential for Baker's cyst?	Exclude phlebitis by using ultrasound
How do you treat Baker's cyst?	NSAIDS and occasionally steroid injection
What is the course of plantar fasciitis?	Resolves spontaneously
What is the course of tarsal tunnel syndrome?	May need surgical release
What is Morton's neuroma?	A painful neuroma between 3rd and 4th toes in which pain gets better after taking the shoe off

Hematology

What are the severe symptoms of anemia?	Shortness of breath and lightheadedness
What is the differential diagnosis for anemia?	Hypoxia, CO poisoning, methemoglobinemia and ischemic heart disease
What disease does show target cells?	Thalassemia
What are the causes of sideroblastic anemia?	ALI(alcohol, lead and INH)
History of blood loss and thrombocytosis does hint to what diagnosis?	Iron deficiency anemia
After CBC what are the best initial tests for iron deficiency anemia?	Iron studies: Fe, TIBC & ferritin
What is the most accurate test for sideroblastic anemia?	Prussian blue
What is the most accurate test for thalassemia?	Hemoglobin electrophoresis
What is the most accurate test for iron deficiency anemia?	Bone marrow biopsy but rarely done
What is the treatment of sideroblastic anemia?	B6 and toxin removal
What is the significance of increased RDW?	Iron deficiency anemia

What do you do if patient has black stool after taking ferrous sulfate and suspicious of occult blood?	Guaiac
What is the diagnosis if ferritin is <15?	Iron deficiency anemia
What is the order of lab findings in iron deficiency anemia?	First ferritin is decreased, then iron is decreased and finally transferrin is increased (TIBC is increased)
What percentage of people with occult GI bleeding is missed when you do sigmoidoscopy?	Misses 40 % of cases
What is the differential for high MCV?	B12, folate, liver disease, alcohol, myelodysplasia, hypothyroidism
What are the main differences between B12 and folate deficiency?	Glossitis, diarrhea, neuropathy. Mild jaundice can be seen due to ineffective erythropoiesis
What is the most common B12 neuropathy?	Peripheral neuropathy
What is the least common B12 neurological deficit?	Dementia
Is B12 neuropathy reversible?	Only if treated early
What are hypersegmented neutrophils?	More than 4
What happens to reticulocyte numbers in B12 deficiency?	It is decreased
What happens to reticulocyte	It is increased

USMLE STEP 3 IN ONE WEEK

numbers in hemolysis?

What changes do we see in LDH, haptoglobin and bilirubin when B12 is deficient?	Normal
When do we see macroovalocytes?	Decrease B12
What reactions do need B12?	Homocysteine to methionine and methylmalonyl CoA to succinyl CoA
When do you see homocysteine level increased?	B12 level and folate level respectively
Why is it that in 30% B12 level is normal?	Transcobalamin is acute phase reactant
What is the next step if B12 is normal?	Methylmalonic acid
When do you see increased level of homocysteine?	Both B12 and folate deficiency can cause that
What is the next step for B12 deficiency etiology?	Antiparietal Ab and anti-intrinsic factor Ab
When do you perform Schilling's test?	Rarely done if Abs are negative
What is the main feature of hemolytic anemia?	Sudden onset of weakness and anemia
What tests do you order for hemolysis?	Smear, LDH, bilirubin, haptoglobin and reticulocytes
What are the main features of intravascular hemolysis?	Abnormal smear(schizocytes, helmet cells), hemosiderinuria and hemoglobinuria

USMLE STEP 3 IN ONE WEEK

What do you see in physical examination of sickle cell anemia?	Physical examination (eyes show retinal infarction, cardiovascular shows flow murmur, splenomegaly, rales and consolidation, extremities ulcer and aseptic necrosis, stroke.
How do you manage sickle cell anemia?	O2, normal saline, antibiotics if fever, morphine, CXR, CBC and smear, reticulocytes, blood culture and urinalysis
What antibiotics are given in sickle cell anemia?	Ceftriaxone or levofloxacin
How dangerous is fever in sickle cell anemia?	Emergency
What are the indications for exchange transfusion in sickle cell anemia?	Retinal infarction, pulmonary infarction, brain infarction and prostate vein infarction
What does cause bone marrow crisis in sickle cell disease?	Decrease folate or parvovirus B19 infection
What is the most accurate test for parvovirus B19?	PCR
How do you treat parvovirus B19 infection?	IVIG or transfusion
With what medications do you send the sickle cell anemia patient home?	Folate, hydroxyurea if more than 4 crisis per year and Pneumococcal vaccine
What are the genotypic variants of sickle cell disease?	SS(sickle cell anemia), AS(trait) and SC

What are the main clinical features of sickle cell trait?	Renal tubular defect called isosthenuria (can't concentrate urine), microscopic hematuria
What clinical feature does SC variant of sickle cell disease have?	Milder version with no painful crisis but renal problems including hematuria and isosthenuria plus UTI
What are the causes of autoimmune hemolytic anemia?	CDL: Connective tissue diseases(SLE and rheumatoid arthritis), Drugs(penicillin, alpha methyldopa, quinidine & lymphoproliferative diseases(CLL and lymphoma)
What is the most accurate test for autoimmune hemolytic anemia?	Coombs
What is the treatment of autoimmune hemolytic anemia?	Steroids, splenectomy, IVIG; note that steroids and splenectomy can control warm Ab(IgG) and not IgM
What are the features of cold induced hemolysis?	Hemolysis happens inside the liver so splenectomy can't help, standard Coombs test is negative but complement test is positive. EBV, mycoplasma and Waldenstrom's macroglobulinemia are the main causes
What is the cause of hemolysis is G6PD deficiency?	Infection, oxidizing drugs(sulfa, primaquine and dapsone) and fava beans

How do you diagnose G6PD deficiency?	Initial test: Heinz bodies and bite cells ; most accurate test is G6PD level if measured when there is no attack for two months
What are the Heinz bodies?	Oxidized Hb precipitates
What is the treatment for G6PD deficiency?	No specific treatment
What are the causes of TTP and HUS?	E Coli O157:H7 , also ticlopidine which is not used anymore
What is the HUS triad?	ART: autoimmune hemolysis, renal problems and thrombocytopenia
What are the main features of TTP?	TTP= ART(autoimmune hemolysis, renal problems and thrombocytopenia) + FN(fever and neurological symptoms)
What is the treatment of TTP or HUS?	Plasmapheresis if it doesn't improve. Don't give antibiotics or platelets
What is the most common cause of death in PNH?	Portal or other large vein thrombosis
What are the two most dangerous complications of PNH?	Aplastic anemia or AML
How do you diagnose PNH?	Decay accelerating factor assay (CD55 and CD59) is the most accurate tests. Sucrose water test, Ham's test are not very accurate test. They activate

	complement
What is the treatment of PNH?	Prednisone
What is the diagnosis if there is shortness of breath and everything is normal?	Brown blood is methemoglobinemia
What drugs can cause methemoglobinemia?	Amyl nitrite, lidocaine and other –caines, dapsone
What is the treatment of methhemoblobinemia?	IV Methylene blue
What are the five main transfusion reactions?	ABO, IgA deficiency, TRALI, febrile non-hemolytic reaction and minor blood groups
What are Auer rods?	AML, they are fused lysosomes with enzymes in them
What type of AML is called M3 and what is the significance of that?	Acute promyelocytic leukemia causing DIC
What is the most important marker of prognosis in AML?	Cytogenetics: if normal (50%) intermediate risk, if t(15;17) or t(8;21) they have favorable outcome
What is the main chemotherapy for M3?	ATRA(all trans retinoic acid) is added to danarubicin and cytarabine which helps the maturation of blast cells
What is the chemotherapy for AML?	Cyclophosphamide and prednisone
What is the chemotherapy for ALL?	Intrathecal methotrexate plus cyclophosphamide and

	prednisone
What is the treatment for leukostasis?	Leukopheresis plus hydroxyurea
What are the main features of leukostasis?	WBC>100,000, blurred vision, CNS and lung symptoms
What are the main features of myelodysplastic syndrome?	Old, pancytopenia, macroovalocytes despite normal B12, Pelger Huet cells(neutrophils with 2 lobes) and small number of blasts
What is the most common cause of death in myelodysplastic syndrome?	Infection
What are the main features of CML?	Splenomegaly, marked leukocytosis and decrease leukocyte alkaline phosphatase plus Philadelphia chromosome
What is the diagnosis if LAP is low and neutrophils are a lot?	CML
What is the most accurate test for CML?	Philadelphia chromosome
What is the pathophysiology of CML?	Protein kinase is stuck in "on position" which is blocked by imatinib(90% remission)
What is the role of bone marrow transplantation in CML?	It is never the initial therapy. Always use imatinib first then BMT
What is one dangerous fate of CML?	Can transform into AML
When do use interferon or hydroxyurea or busulfan in CML?	Never

USMLE STEP 3 IN ONE WEEK

What is the main feature of CLL? — Normal appearing lymphocytes in over 50 people

What is the best initial test for CLL? — Blood smear showing smudge cells

What are the stages of CLL? — Stage 0 is increase WBC, stage 1 is adenopathy, stage 2 is splenomegaly, stage 3 is anemia and stage 4 is thrombocytopenia. Stage 0 and 1 need no treatment, stage 2,3 and 4 can benefit from fludarabine

What are the main features of hairy cell leukemia? — Middle age, massive splenomegaly, pancytopenia, TRAP(a form of acid phosphatase) shows hairy cells

How do you treat hairy cell leukemia? — Cladribine/ 2-CDA

What are the main features of myelofibrosis? — Pancytopenia plus massive splenomegaly, tear drop cells, dry tap and no treatment

What is the main diagnostic clue for polycythemia vera? — Low erythropoietin level and high hematocrit

What is anagrelide for? — Treatment of thrombocytosis

How do you treat polycythemia vera? — PAHA: phlebotomy, aspirin, hydroxyurea and anagrelide

What is the treatment of essential thrombocytosis? — AHA: aspirin, anagrelide and hydroxyurea

What is the main prognostic factor in multiple myeloma? — Beta2 microglobulin

USMLE STEP 3 IN ONE WEEK

What is the most accurate test for multiple myeloma?	Bone marrow biopsy
What is the treatment for multiple myeloma?	If young and advance disease autologous bone marrow transplantation otherwise use MST: melphalan, steroids and thalidomide(TNF inhibitor)
What is the diagnosis in a patient >70 with high IgG and nothing else?	MGUS and there is no need for treatment
How do you diagnose Waldenstrom's macroglobulinemia?	Increase serum viscosity and SPEP
What is the treatment for Waldenstrom's?	Plasmapheresis, fludarabine and chlorambucil
What is the treatment for aplastic anemia?	>50 ATG plus cyclosporine ; <50 BM transplantation if there is a match otherwise ATG and cyclosporine
What is the best initial test for lymphoma?	Excisional biopsy
What are the staging tests for lymphoma?	CXR, CT with contrast and BM biopsy
What is the treatment for stage I and II lymphoma?	Radiation
What is the treatment for stage III and IV lymphoma?	ABVC or CHOP; if CD20 positive add rituximab to CHOP
vWF can bind to what structures?	Only binds collagen, platelets and heparin
Platelet type bleeding and normal	Von Willibrand disease

USMLE STEP 3 IN ONE WEEK

platelet count is seen in what disease?

What is the best initial test in vWD?	Bleeding time
What is ristocetin function assay?	Ristocetin is like naked collagen and causes platelet agglutination if vWF is present in large amount
What is the most accurate test in vWD?	Ristocetin and vWF level. Ristocetin shows if vWF works normally
What changes are seen in factor VIII level in vWD?	F VIII is decreased and APTT is prolonged in 50%
What is the treatment of vWD?	Vasopressin and F VIII replacement
Why does vWD cause F VIII deficiency?	vWF is a carrier for F VIII and without it the half-life is decreased
What is aPTT?	PLP plus calcium and kaolin
What is PT?	Tissue factor and calcium
What is INR?	INR is the ratio of patient PT to normal PT (base on normal distribution graph)
When do you give IVIG in ITP?	If platelets are <20 000 in ITP
What is the treatment of ITP if platelets are >50 000?	No treatment
What is the treatment of ITP if platelets are between 20 to 50	Prednisone

thousands?

What is the diagnosis if platelet count is normal, vWF and ristocetin are normal and there is platelet type bleeding?	Renal disease should be ruled out (uremia causes degranulation problem)
What is the diagnosis if mixing studies can't correct aPTT?	Factor inhibiting Ab or antiphospholipid or heparin is present
What is the best initial treatment for uremia induced platelet dysfunction?	vasopressin
What is the treatment of F XI deficiency?	Fresh frozen plasma
What is the mechanism of action of heparin?	Antithrombin III inhibitor becomes inactive
What is HIT (heparin induced thrombocytopenia?	Allergic reaction to heparin destroys platelets and causes thrombosis
What is the best initial test for HIT?	Antiplatelet Ab, platelet factor 4 Ab
What is the treatment for HIT?	Stop heparin (for life) and use thrombin inhibitors like argatroban or lepirudin; start warfarin only if platelets >150000
What is the most common thrombophilia?	Factor V Leiden mutation makes it resistant to protein C and S
How do you treat factor V Leiden?	Warfarin for the rest of their lives (start heparin for the first

	few days until warfarin starts working)
What are other types of thrombophilia?	Low protein C and S, lupus anticoagulant and decrease antithrombin
What happens if antithrombin III is deficient?	Resistance to heparin
What is the mechanism of lupus anticoagulant/anticardiolipin Ab/antiphospholipid Ab?	Venous thrombosis because autoantibodies bind to cells and phospholipids of cell membrane
What test is used for diagnosis of lupus anticoagulant?	Russell's viper venom time is prolonged
What is the treatment for lupus anticoagulant?	Heparin and warfarin

Gastrointestinal Diseases

What are the main differences between orophayngeal dysphagia and esophageal?	Esophageal is not associated with initiating swallowing and is felt in upper chest however orophayngeal is associated with coughing, drooling and sometimes ear pain
What is the first initial test for dysphagia?	Barium study
What is the most accurate test for achalasia?	Manometery shows absence of peristalsis and increased LES pressure(failure to relax)
How do you treat achalasia?	Balloon dilation, botulinum toxin injection and surgery
If suspicious of esophageal cancer, what is the best initial test?	Endoscopy
What is Plummer-Vinson syndrome?	Proximal web which increases chance of squamous cell carcinoma
Where is Schatzki ring?	Distal esophagus
What is the diagnosis of dysphagia plus horrible bad breath?	Zenker's diverticulum (don't scope them)
What is the main feature of diffuse esophageal spasm?	Always pain; also manometry shows increased pressure across esophagus, corkscrew shape in barium meal, treat with Ca channel blockers

Can you see ST elevation in Prinzmetal angina?	Yes
What is the next step in management of esophagitis?	If HIV negative scope them; if HIV positive and CD4<100 give fluconazole for both diagnosis and treatment. If no response scope them
What percentage of HIV patients has candida esophagitis?	>90%
What are other common causes of esophagitis?	Doxycycline, alendronate(remain upright for 30 minutes after drinking a lot of water)
How do you treat Mallory-Weiss tear?	Nothing or epinephrine injection
What is the first line of management for GERD?	PPI is both diagnostic and therapeutic
What other symptoms are seen in GERD?	Chronic cough, hoarseness, wheezing, metallic taste and sore throat
What percentage of patients with chronic cough has GERD?	20%
How do you diagnose GERD?	PPI, 24h pH monitoring
When do people with GERD need endoscopy?	BAD-W: blood in stool, anemia, dysphagia and weight loss
How do you treat GERD?	Lifestyle modification, PPI, H2 blockers only if PPI is not available. If all fails surgery is the choice. Nissen fundoplication or endoscopically narrowing LES

USMLE STEP 3 IN ONE WEEK

How do you diagnose Barrett's esophagus? Though the color of mucosa is different biopsy is needed

What are the indications for biopsy in GERD?
1. BAD-W (blood in stool, anemia, dysphagia & weight loss)
2. >5 years of esophagitis
3. If Barrett's give PPI and every 2-3 year endoscopy
4. If low grade dysplasia scope them every 3-6 months
5. If high grade dysplasia do esophagectomy

How do you manage dyspepsia? If associated with GERD symptoms treat with PPI
If history of NSAIDS use stop medication
In other cases if more than 45 endoscopy is needed and if younger H. pylori testing

What are the adverse effects of PPI? Osteoporosis (suppresses Ca absorption), C. diff, decrease Fe, B12 and Mg absorption, interaction with clopidogrel (decrease its effect)

What is the most common cause of epigastric discomfort? Non-ulcer dyspepsia

How do you diagnose non-ulcer dyspepsia? It is diagnosis of exclusion

What is the benefit of treating H. pylori in non-ulcer dyspepsia? No proven benefit in treating H. pylori

What is the treatment of non-ulcer dyspepsia? H2 blockers, liquid antacid and PPI

What is the relationship between Crohn's causes peptic ulcer

Crohn's and peptic ulcer?

How do you diagnose H. pylori infection?	Biopsy is the most accurate Serology is very sensitive so negative test excludes it Breath test and Stool Ag is performed if serology is positive
When do you treat H. pylori infection?	Only if it is associated with symptoms or there is gastritis or peptic ulcer
What is the treatment of H. pylori infection?	Amoxicillin plus clarithromycin and PPI
What is the treatment of H. pylori if triple therapy fails?	Metronidazole, tetracycline, bismuth plus PPI
What if the second line of treatment for H. pylori is failing?	Suspect Zollinger-Ellison's syndrome
What are the indications of stress ulcer prophylaxis?	Head trauma, Intubation and mechanical ventilation, burns, coagulopathy and steroid use
What do you do if there is no gastritis or ulcer but H. pylori is present?	Don't treat for H. pylori
When do you confirm H. pylori eradication?	A urea breath test 4 weeks after therapy
What is the best initial test for Zollinger-Ellison?	Gastrin level and gastric acid output
What is the differential for hypergastrinemia?	Any H2 blocker or PPI can do that
When do we check for Zollinger-Ellison?	>1 cm ulcer, multiple ulcers, recurrent or persistent H. pylori despite treatment, distal location of

	ulcers
What diagnostic modalities do you use for Zollinger-Ellison if both gastrin level and acid output are high?	Endoscopic ultrasound is more sensitive than regular ultrasound; nuclear somatostatin scan shows increase number of receptors for somatostatin; secretin suppression test
What is the effect of IV secretin test?	Secretin decreases gastrin and acid output level but not in Zollinger-Ellison
What is the treatment of Zollinger-Ellison?	If local surgery; if metastatic lifelong PPI
What is the next step if Zollinger-Ellison and hypercalcemia happen together?	Rule out MEN syndrome
What biliary disease is seen with inflammatory bowel diseases?	Sclerosing cholangitis
What is the screening for IBD >10 years?	Yearly endoscopy
Why do we see hypocalcemia in Crohn's?	Malabsorption
Which IBD shoes calcium oxalate and cholesterol stones?	Crohn's
How do you diagnose IBD?	Scope or barium studies and blood tests
What blood tests are important in differentiating Crohn's from UC?	Crohn's ANCA and Ulcerative colitis pANCA positive

What is the best initial treatment for IBD?	Mesalamine
What is the best Tx for acute exacerbation of IBD?	Budesonide (for acute exacerbation) ; it has very high first pass effect
How do we treat IBD recurrence after steroids? How do you treat fistulas in IBD?	Azathioprine or 6-mercaptopurine Infliximab (PPD before administering)
How do you treat perianal diseases of IBD?	Ciprofloxacin plus metronidazole
IBD treatment if existed for a long time and there is complications?	Surgery
What side effects do limit use of sulfasalazine?	Rash, hemolysis, interstitial nephritis
How do you classify diarrhea?	Acute and chronic; acute is inflammatory or non-inflammatory, chronic can be osmotic, secretory, inflammatory, malabsorption, motility disorders, infection and factitious
What is the workup for inflammatory diarrhea?	If there is blood it is inflammatory, if no blood but there is WBC it is inflammatory, if no blood and no WBC but culture is positive it is inflammatory
What are the causes for infectious diarrhea?	Campylobacter, Salmonella, Vibrio parahemolyticus, Vibrio vulnificus, E coli, Shigella, Yersinia and amoeba
What is the most common cause of gateroenteritis?	Norwalk virus
What is the most common cause	Campylobacter

of food poisoning?

What are the complications of Campylobacter infection?	Guillain-Barre syndrome and arthritis
What is the source of Vibrio parahemolyticus food poisoning?	Seafood
What are the types of E coli infection?	ETEC, EIEC, O157:H7
What are the main features of Vibrio vulnificus food poisoning?	Liver and skin diseases
How do you get Yersinia enterocolitis?	Rodents, pork meat
What are the indications for antibiotic therapy in infectious diarrhea?	Fever, abdominal pain, blood in stool and low blood pressure
How do you diagnose Giardiosis?	ELISA stool for Ag
What is the source of Bacillus cereus infection?	Fried rice (it resolves spontaneously)
How do you teat cryptosporidiosis?	No proven treatment but in HIV patients treat HIV and add paromomycin
How do you diagnose cryptosporidiosis?	CD4<100 and modified acid fast staining
What is scombroid?	Histamine release from infected tuna, mackerel and mahi mahi; treat with antihistaminic
How do you diagnose C. difficile infection?	Stool toxin assay
What are the lab abnormalities for severe C. diff?	wBC>15000 Cr >1.5 times normal

	Albumin <2.5
When do you use vancomycin in the treatment of C. difficile infection?	Only if you have tried metronidazole twice
What are the main features of carcinoid?	Flushing and low blood pressure plus increased urinary 5HIAA
What is the treatment of carcinoid?	Octreotide
How do you diagnose fat malabsorption?	Stool fat staining with Sudan black; also 72h fat in stool is the most sensitive
What are the differentials for fat malabsorption?	Whipple's, tropical sprue, chronic pancreatitis and celiac disease
How do we have oxalate stones in malabsorption syndromes?	Fat malabsorption causes increased absorption of oxalates
What are the main problems of vitamin deficiency in malabsorption syndromes?	Vitamin K deficiency increases PT and causes bleeding; Vitamin B12 deficiency causes megaloblastic anemia and vitamin D deficiency causes osteoporosis
What three antibodies are seen in celiac disease?	Anti-tissue transglutaminase is the best initial test; antigliadin and antiendomysial antibodies
What is the most accurate test for celiac disease?	Biopsy is always necessary
What is the diagnosis if a patient with celiac disease is on gluten free diet and still has symptoms?	Intestinal lymphoma must be ruled out in a case of refractory celiac disease
What is the use of D-xylose test?	Rarely used for malabsorption and it is not specific; just shows damage to villous lining

USMLE STEP 3 IN ONE WEEK

What is the treatment for Whipple's and tropical sprue?	6 months for tropical sprue and one year for Whipple disease (tetracycline plus Bactrim)
What is the most accurate test for tropical sprue and Whipple's?	Biopsy shoes PAS positive microorganisms in Whipple and show the bacteria for tropical sprue, also PCR for Tropheryema whipplei
What are the levels of amylase and lipase in chronic pancreatitis?	Amylase and lipase are normal because they are finished and pancreas is burnt out
What is the best initial test for chronic pancreatitis?	Abdominal X-ray or CT scan of abdomen
What is the most accurate test for chronic pancreatitis?	Secretin stimulation test fails to produce profuse bicarbonate
What are the levels of D-xylose, folate and Fe in chronic pancreatitis?	Normal
What is irritable bowel syndrome?	Alternating diarrhea and constipation plus abdominal pain relieved by defecation which is less at night and no blood, fever or weight loss
How do you diagnose IBS?	Guaiac, WBC, ova, culture, colonoscopy and CT abdomen must be negative
What is the treatment for IBS?	FAT: fiber, antispasmodics, tricyclic antidepressants
What is the use of tricyclic antidepressants in IBS?	They are anticholinergic, antineuropathic and antidepressant
What are the routine	Every 10 years start at 50 except for:

colonoscopy recommendations?	- 1st degree less than 60 or 2 first degree at any age start at 40 or 10 years younger than relative - people with tubular adenoma which need every 3-5 years - If >10 adenoma repeat every 1-2 year - If >2 cm sessile polyp removed by piecemeal every 2-6 months
What are the criteria for Lynch syndrome (HNPCC)?	3,2,1 rule: 3 family members, 2 generation and 1 premature(less than 50). They must have colonoscopy after 25 every 1-2 year
What is Gardner's syndrome?	Osteoma and colonic polyps
What is Peutz-Jegher syndrome?	Lip melanosis and colonic polyps
What kind of polyps do you see in juvenile polyps?	Hamartomatous
How do you manage dysplastic polyps?	colonoscopy every 3-5 years
What is the indication of colonoscopy in diverticular diseases?	it is contraindicated in diverticulitis but in diverticulosis it is the most accurate test
What is the best test for diverticulosis?	CT
What is the treatment of diverticulitis?	Metronidazole plus ciprofloxacin
How much blood is needed for black stool?	100 ml of blood

USMLE STEP 3 IN ONE WEEK

How much blood is needed for heme positive stool?	10 ml of blood
How much blood loss needed for BP<100 or PR>100?	1/3 of blood loss
What is orthostatic hypotension?	>20 mmHg drop and > 10 beat increase
What is the indication of packed RBC infusion?	Hematocrit <30 in old and <20-25 in yonder patients with no heart diseases
Hwo do you mange INR which is more than therapeutic level but is less than 5?	Hold warfarin for 2 days and decrease the dose afterward until it is normal
How do you manage INR which is more than 9?	Hold warfarin, give oral vitamin K; you can also do the same thing if INR is 5-9 if the risk of bleeding is high
What do you give FFP and why?	If there is serious bleeding V.K is too slow to act
What is the danger of IV vitamin K?	Anaphylaxis
When do you give platelets?	<50 000 if bleeding or surgery
What is the most common cause of death in GI bleeding?	MI because myocardium doesn't get enough blood
When do you use iced saline lavage?	Never
What are the most important measures of severity of BI bleeding?	BP and HR
What happens if you give too	Hypoxia because of dilution. Give

much fluid in GI bleeding?	oxygen
What do you have to do before endoscopy in GI bleeding?	Correct anemia, platelets and coagulopathy
What percentage of GI bleeding stops without scope?	80%
What do you do if ulcer is present in GI bleeding?	Add PPI
What 3 disease need octreotide?	Variceal bleeding, carcinoid and acromegaly
What is the treatment of variceal bleeding?	Octreotide, endoscopy banding and TIPS (hepatic encephalopathy can be a complication)
What are the causes of hepatic encephalopathy?	Low volume, low O2, low glucose, low K, GI bleeding, SBP
When do you use Blackmore balloon?	Rarely performed. Just to stop bleeding to allow shunt
What are the causes of upper GI bleeding?	In order of frequency: peptic ulcer, gastritis, varices, cancer
When do you transfuse in upper GI bleeding?	If Hb is <7 unless there is other risk factors e.g. coronary artery disease
What are the causes of lower GI bleeding?	In order of frequency: angiodysplasia, diverticulosis, IBD, cancer and polyps, ischemic colitis
What diseases are associated with angiodysplasia?	Aortic stenosis and ESRD
How do you diagnose GI bleeding?	Scope them and if negative use technetium labeled RBC. If positive use angiography preoperatively. If negative use capsule endoscopy (disadvantage is no possibility for biopsy)

USMLE STEP 3 IN ONE WEEK

How do you diagnose acute mesenteric ischemia?

Pain out of proportion in physical exam; amylase is increased, metabolic acidosis. Angiography is the most accurate test.(if untreated they die)

What are the differentials for constipation?

Dehydration, Ca channel blockers, narcotics, hypothyroidism, diabetes, Fe, anticholinergics, cancer and immobility. Treatment is hydration and docusate

How do you treat chronic constipation if fluid and fiber didn't help?

BOSS: bulk forming, osmotic, stimulants and saline agents

What are the main causes of black stool?

Blood or Fe (heme negative)

What is the clue in dumping syndrome?

Decreased BP

What is the treatment of dumping syndrome?

Small frequent meals

What are the causes of acute pancreatitis?

GA HIT ME : gallstone, alcohol, hyperlipidemia, infection, trauma, medications and ERCP. Medications are: thiazides, azathioprine, didanosine and Stavudine, valproate, sulfasalazine

How do you diagnose acute pancreatitis?

Amylase, lipase and CT

What are the signs of severe pancreatitis?

Hyperglycemia, hypocalcemia, hypotension, hypoxia, hypovolemia, leukocytosis and metabolic acidosis

What is the best criteria for

APACHE II which has 12 variables and

severity of pancreatitis?	if it is 8 or higher it is severe Variables include 4 vital signs, Na, K, Glasgow coma scale, WBC, Cr, Hct, A-a difference, pH Ranson's has low positive predictive value
When do you do ERCP?	Dilation of CBD and no pancreatic mass
What is the marker of severity in acute pancreatitis?	Dilation of CBD and no pancreatic mass
What is the marker of severity in acute pancreatitis?	Urine trypsinogen activation peptide
What is the initial treatment of acute pancreatitis?	NPO, fluid and pain killer
What pain killers are used for acute pancreatitis?	Meperidine or morphine (sphincter of Oddi spasm isn't a concern anymore)
How does CT help with the management of acute pancreatitis?	CT shows less than 30% necrosis treat conservatively. If it shows >30% necrosis give imipenem and do CT guided biopsy; if necrotic pancreas is seen on biopsy do surgical debridement
How long do you need for chronic hepatitis?	More than 6 months
How do you interpret Hep B Ags and Abs?	HBsAg positive means acute or chronic disease HBeAg positive means acute viral replication HBsAb means vaccination or recovered HBcAb means recovered or window period

How do you evaluate hepatitis C severity and activity?	PCR shows viral replication but biopsy is needed for accurate evaluation of severity
What is the damage after 10 years of viral replication in hepatitis C?	Very little liver damage
When do you start treating Hepatitis C with ribavirin and interferon?	When biopsy shows at least moderate inflammation
What is the treatment of chronic hepatitis B?	Lamivudine, entecavir, telbivudine, interferon alpha and adefovir
How do you treat hepatitis B needle injury?	Hep B immunoglobulins and vaccination
Is there any post exposure treatment for hepatitis C?	None
What are the signs and symptoms of cirrhosis?	Edema, palmar erythema, splenomegaly, anemia, thrombocytopenia, coagulopathy (V.K is low), PT is increased, telangiectasia, esophageal varices, hepatorenal syndrome, encephalopathy, ascites, spontaneous bacterial peritonitis
How do you treat cirrhosis?	Spironolactone and diuretics, FeSo4, folate, V.K, FFP, variceal banding, transfusion, albumin plus vasopressin(used in hepatorenal), antibiotics, lactulose (short chain fatty acids make H+ which makes NH4+ from NH3 which can't be absorbed

USMLE STEP 3 IN ONE WEEK

When do you tap ascites?	New ascites or if pain/tenderness/fever is there.
What is SAAG and its importance?	Serum/ ascites albumin gradient; if it is >1.1 it is portal HTN or CHF. If it is <1.1 it is exudate.
What is the treatment for spontaneous bacterial peritonitis?	Cefotaxime or ceftriaxone
How do you diagnose alcoholic cirrhosis?	Diagnosis of exclusion but AST/ALT>2 helps. Also alkaline phosphatase rarely is more than three times.
What are the main features of primary biliary cirrhosis?	Normal bilirubin initially, increased alkaline phosphatase; AMA (most accurate test) and IgM are increased. Malabsorption of vitamin D causes osteoporosis
What is the treatment of PBC?	Ursodeoxycholic acid (suppresses immune response)
How do you diagnose primary sclerosing cholangitis?	ERCP shows beading(most accurate test), increased ASMA, ANCA and bilirubin
What is the treatment of PSC?	Ursodeoxycholic
What is the initial best test for Wilson's disease?	Slit lamp
What kind of anemia is seen in Wilson's?	Hemolytic anemia
How do you treat Wilson's	Penicillamine, zinc and trientine

disease?

What are the main features of hemochromatosis?

Skin: pigmentation; pituitary: panhypopituitarism; liver cirrhosis and hepatocellular carcinoma; joints: pseudogout
pancreas

What is the best initial test for hemochromatosis?

Iron studies: Fe, ferritin & saturation (increased), TIBC (decreased)

What is the most accurate test for hemochromatosis?

Biopsy; MRI plus genetic testing can replace biopsy

How do you treat hemochromatosis?

Phlebotomy

What are the main features of autoimmune hepatitis?

Young female with other autoimmune diseases like ITP, Coombs positive, thyroiditis, with positive ASMA (anti-smooth muscle Ab) , ANA, SPEP showing gammapathy, liver and kidney microsomal Ab

What are the main features of autoimmune hepatitis?
What is the most accurate test for diagnosis of autoimmune hepatitis?

ANA, anti smooth muscle Ab, history of autoimmune diseases
Biopsy; treatment is prednisone

What are the main features of non-alcoholic steatohepatitis (NASH)?

ALT>AST, treat underlying disease e.g. Obesity, hyperlipidemia or diabetes

What is pylephlebitis?

Infectious thrombosis of portal vein usually a complication of ruptured

USMLE STEP 3 IN ONE WEEK

appendix

Neurology

What risk factor is the most important in stroke?	hypertension
What is TIA?	Transient ischemic attack which is around 1-2 hours and never >24h; it is never hemorrhagic
What is stroke?	>24h with permanent deficit; 80% is ischemic and 20% is hemorrhagic
What is the first test before giving any oral medications including statins?	Swallowing studies
How high blood pressure can be in stroke?	185/105
Why do we give LMWH in ischemic stroke patiens?	To prevent DVT
What are the main features of anterior cerebral artery stroke?	Personality changes, urinary incontinence and profound lower extremity weakness (upper is mild)
What are the main features of middle cerebral artery stroke?	Profound upper limb impairment, aphasia, apraxia if nondominant lobe (neglect), eyes deviate towards the lesion
What are the main features of posterior cerebral artery stroke?	Contralateral homonymous hemianopia with macular sparing, prosopagnosia (can't recognize faces)
What are the main features of vertebrobasilar artery system stroke?	Vertigo, vomiting, vertical nystagmus, walking problems (ataxia), drop attacks, dysarthria, sensory changes of the face

USMLE STEP 3 IN ONE WEEK

What are the main features of lacunar infarct?	Absence of cortical deficit, basal ganglia signs e.g. Parkinsonism; ataxia, sensory deficit and hemiparesis
How do you differentiate clinically brain stem lesions and corticothalamic lesions?	Brain stem lesion involve ipsilateral face while corticothalamic lesions involve contralateral face
What are the main features of lateral medullary syndrome?	Wallengberg syndrome has Verterbral artery lesions, Vestibulocochlear signs including Vertigo; Dysphagia, Dysarthria, Dysphonia,
What are the differences between MRI and CT in stroke?	MRI >95% accurate in 24h, CT >95% accurate in 3-5 days
What is the window period for tPA in stroke?	3-4.5 hours
What are the contraindications for tPA?	Active bleeding or surgery (last 6 weeks), Hx of hemorrhagic stroke, stroke within one year, bleeding disorders, traumatic CPR in the last 3 weeks, cerebral trauma in the last 6 months, cerebral mass or neoplasm, suspicious aortic dissection, BP 185/110
How do you treat stroke?	EKG, Echocardiography, Holter's monitor, carotid artery Doppler, if <50 do: ESR, VDRL, RPR, ANA, anti- DS DNA, protein C,S, factor V Leiden and antiphospholipid antibody
What is the further management of stroke?	Diabetes and hypertension control
What is the diagnosis if there is DVT and embolic stroke?	Paradoxical embolism

USMLE STEP 3 IN ONE WEEK

When is endartrectomy indicated?	Systolic less than 130, diastolic less than 80, LDL less than 100, tight glycemic control
How do you treat status epilepticus?	Lorazepam (Ativan), after 10-20 minutes fosphenytoin, after 10-20 minutes phenobarbital, after 10-20 minutes pentobarbital
What are the initial diagnostic tests for seizure?	Electrolytes, chemistry, if CT normal do MRI, urine toxicology
What further test do you order for seizure?	EEG
Can potassium disorders cause seizure?	Never
When do you treat even one seizure as epilepsy?	Strong family history, EEG abnormal and status epilepticus requiring benzodiazepines for treatment
What are the first line antiepileptics?	Levetriacetam, phenytoin, valproate & carbamazepine
What are the second line antiepileptics?	Gabapantine or phenobarbital
What is the best treatment for absence seizure?	Ethosuximide
When do you use lamotrigine and what is the most dangerous side effect?	Equal to first line but be careful of Steven Johnson's syndrome
What cognitive changes do you see in Parkinson's disease?	Normal cognition and memory however almost half of them have major depressive disorder
What is the treatment for	>60 amantadine, <60 anticholinergics e.g.

mild Parkinson's?	Benztropine or trihexylphenidate
What is the treatment for moderate Parkinson's?	Sinemet(L-DOPA plus carbidopa), selegiline and one of dopamine receptor agonists: pramipaxole, cabergoline or ropinerole
What is the treatment for severe Parkinson's?	Bromocriptine, pramipaxole/cabergoline/ropinerole, selegiline
How do you treat tremor?	Amantadine if Parkinson, treat the underlying disease for intention tremor ; propranolol for essential tremor
What are the tests necessary before diagnosing multiple sclerosis?	VDRL, B12, TSH, CT scan and MRI
How do you treat multiple sclerosis?	Acute needs steroids, baclofen or tizanidine used for spasticity, beta interferon, natalizumab
What are the late manifestations of Alzheimer's?	Apathy and imprecise speech
What is the only abnormality seen on Alzheimer's workup?	CT shows diffuse symmetrical atrophy
How do you treat Alzheimer's?	Galantamine, rivastigmine, donepezil and memantine
What is the mechanism of action of memantine?	Blocks NMDA receptor
What are the main features of Pick's disease?	Frontotemporal atrophy, personality changes before dementia; treatment same as Alzheimer's

USMLE STEP 3 IN ONE WEEK

What is Lewy body dementia?

It is dementia, parkinsonism, visual hallucination, fluctuation of disease, severe reaction to neuroleptics
It should be differentiated from Parkinson's dementia

How do you treat Lewy body dementia?

Treatment of Alzheimer's and Parkinson's together

What is CJD disease?

Prion is the cause, rapid progressive dementia, myoclonus, 14-3-3 protein in CSF; abnormal EEG and no need for biopsy

What are the main features of normal pressure hydrocephalus?

WWW: wide gait (ataxia); wet (urinary incontinence); weird (dementia)

How do you diagnose normal pressure hydrocephalus?

CT and LP (normal pressure)

How do you treat normal pressure hydrocephalus?

LP removal of CSF and if it responds the main treatment i.e. Shunt will be effective

What percentage of migraine is bilateral?

40%

What is the indication of CT/MRI in headache?

>40, sudden severe and neurological deficit, personality changes, systemic signs

What is the treatment for migraine?

Dark and quiet room, analgesics, sumatriptan and ergotamine

What is the migraine prophylaxis?

If > 3 attacks in a month or severely disabling usecalcium channel blockers (esp. verapamil), beta blockers, tricyclic antidepressants or SSRI

What is the prophylactic

None

treatment for cluster headache?	
How do you treat cluster headache?	100% O2, steroids, sumatriptan
Can cluster headache be bilateral?	Never
What are the main features of pseudotumor cerebri?	Female, double vision, headache, papilledema, CN VI palsy, CT/MRI normal, LP shows high opening pressure
What medications do cause pseudotumor cerebri?	V.A derivatives, tetracyclines, danazol, tamoxifen and steroids, Lithium
What is the treatment of pseudotumor cerebri?	Acetazolamide, weight loss, steroids and stop V.A if the cause
What is the one test that generally all patients with vertigo should have?	MRI of the auditory canal
What are the causes of vertigo?	Meniere's disease (tinnitus, vertigo & hearing loss), benign positional vertigo, acoustic neuroma, perilymph fistula and vestibular neuronitis
What is the treatment for BPV or vestibular neuronitis or labyrinthitis?	Meclizine
What is the treatment for Meniere's disease?	Salt restriction and diuretics
How do you differentiate Meniere's disease and labyrinthitis?	Meniere's is chronic and labyrinthitis is acute but both have tinnitus, hearing loss and vertigo
What are the main features	Tinnitus, hearing loss, vertigo and ataxia

of acoustic neuroma?

What are the main features of Wernicke encephalopathy and Korsakoff psychosis?	Chronic alcohol use, confusion, confabulation, ataxia, nystagmus, gaze palsy and memory loss
How do you treat Wernicke Korsakoff - psychosis?	B1 before glucose (if glucose is given first B1 may be used for glucose metabolism)
Which test is usually done before LP in CNS infection?	CT
What are the indications of CT before LP?	Papilledema, seizure, altered level of consciousness, focal neurological deficit, history of CNS diseases and significant delay in lumbar puncture performance
What are the main features of Parinaud's syndrome?	Upward gaze paly, ataxia, headache and hydrocephalus
What do you do in CNS infection before doing CT and LP?	Do culture and start antibiotics
What is the best initial test for meningitis?	CSF cell count; if thousand neutrophils then start ceftriaxone + vancomycin + steroids
What are the main features of CSF analysis?	G stain (60% positive), glucose (must be <60% of blood level), protein (if normal bacterial meningitis is ruled out and cell count
What bacteria are seen on G stain of CSF?	Pneumococcus, Neisseria, Hemophilus and Listeria
What are the main features of Cryptococcus meningitis?	CD4 < 100 India ink is the best initial test Cryptococcus Ag testing is the most accurate test

USMLE STEP 3 IN ONE WEEK

How do you treat Cryptococcus meningitis?	Amphotericin followed by life time fluconazole unless CD4 is raised
What are the main features of Rocky Mountain spotted fever?	Rash on wrist and ankle, fever before rash, serology and treatment is doxycycline
What is the treatment for TB meningitis?	RIPES: RIPE (rifampin, INH, pyrazinamide and ethambutol) and steroids; RIPE is continued for a year
What is the Listeria meningitis coverage?	Ampicillin is added to ceftriaxone and vancomycin
What is the Listeria meningitis prophylaxis?	Rifampin or ciprofloxacin is given to close contact (kissing or sharing utensils)
What are the main features of encephalitis?	Fever + confusion develops very fast; almost always herpes simplex virus is the cause
How do you diagnose encephalitis?	CT is the best initial test to rule out other causes; LP & PCR of CSF, no need for brain biopsy
What is the treatment of encephalitis?	Acyclovir and if resistant use foscarnet
What is the management of fever +headache + focal neurological deficit?	Contrast CT; if positive it is either tumor or abscess
What is the next step in brain abscess?	If HIV negative do biopsy; if HIV positive treat for 2 weeks with pyrimethamine and sulfadiazine if resolves nor further tests needed

What is the treatment of neurocysticercosis?	Albendazole + steroids
What are the main features of postconcussive syndrome?	Headache, confusion, problems with concentration, anxiety and sleep problems
What is the treatment of head trauma?	Concussion: observe Contusion: mostly none Epi and subdural hematoma: surgery if large Increased ICP: hyperventilate, mannitol and intubation to keep CO2<25-30; steroids Ulcer prophylaxis in head trauma is needed
What are the indications of CT in head trauma?	Altered mental status FND GCS abnormal Basilar skull fracture signs Bleeding diathesis
What are the main features of subarachnoid hemorrhage?	Meningismus, loss of consciousness and absent of fever
What do you do if CT is positive in SAH?	No need for LP; if negative do LP
How do you differentiate traumatic tap from SAH? What result of LP is considered positive for infection?	If the WBC/RBC ratio is similar to blood it is traumatic tap (1:1000) If WBC/RBC is > 1/500 it is considered infection
What is the treatment of SAH?	Nimodipine, angiography, surgery (clip or embolization), shunt
What is the prognosis of rebleed in SAH if we don't do surgery?	50% die

What is the major difference between SAH of PCA and PICA?	PICA shows ataxia and PCA shows CN III palsy
What are the clinical features of syringomyelia?	Hand and shoulder loss of spinothalamic tract bilaterally; diagnose with MRI
What are the causes of syringomyelia?	Trauma, tumor and congenital
What is the treatment of syringomyelia?	Surgery
What is the most urgent treatment of cod compression?	Steroids and maybe surgery
What are the causes of cord compression?	Bone: fracture, dislocation, spondylosis and abnormal growth; blood (hematoma), tumor (usually metastasis), disc herniation
What is the treatment of spinal cord abscess?	Oxacillin, nafcillin and maybe surgery
What are the signs of anterior spinal artery occlusion?	Loss of pain and temperature (intact vibration and sense of position)
What is Brown-Sequard syndrome?	Lateral knife trauma can cause loss of ipsilateral position and vibration + contralateral spinothalamic
What is the diagnosis of fever, focal spinal pain and focal neurological deficit with high ESR and CRP?	Spinal epidural abscess which needs immediate surgical intervention
What is the cause of dyspnea in ALS?	Involvement of diaphragm
What is the treatment of amyotrophic lateral	Riluzole blocks accumulation of glutamate

USMLE STEP 3 IN ONE WEEK

sclerosis?

What is Saturday night palsy?	Wrist drop due to radial nerve palsy
What kind of nerve damage is seen with high boots?	Peroneal nerve palsy
What is the treatment of Bell's palsy?	Acyclovir and steroids
How do you treat reflex sympathetic dystrophy?	Gabapantine, NSAIDS, surgical block and sympathectomy
What are the causes of restless syndrome?	Mostly is idiopathic however secondary causes are DUMPIMP (DM, Uremia, MS, Parkinson's, iron deficiency anemia, medications and pregnancy
How do you treat restless leg syndrome?	1st line: Pramipaxole or ropinerole 2nd line: gabapentin , enacarbin
What is the treatment of Guillain Barre syndrome?	Peak inspiratory pressure, IVIG or plasmapheresis
How do you diagnose myasthenia gravis?	Clinical diagnosis and acetylcholine receptor Ab
What is the treatment of myasthenia gravis?	Pyridostigmine, neostigmine, thymectomy, prednisone, AC
What is the treatment of myasthenia gravis in order?	First neostigmine and if it doesn't work thymectomy and if it doesn't work steroids and if it doesn't stop it switch to azathioprine and cyclophosphamide

Nephrology

What are the clues to renal failure of very short duration?	Normal kidney size, normal hematocrit, normal calcium level
How long does it take for hemoglobin to go down in renal failure?	2 weeks because of short half-life of erythropoietin
What are the causes of pre-renal azotemia?	Hypotension, hypovolemia renal artery stenosis, decreased oncotic pressure (low albumin e.g. Hepatorenal syndrome), CHF & constrictive pericarditis
How do you diagnose pre-renal azotemia?	BUN/Cr > 15 or 20 Fractional excretion of Na(FENa) <1% Urinary sodium < 20 (aldosterone effect) Urine osmolality >500
What do you have to order for all the renal causes of renal failure?	U/A, ultrasound, chemistry
What do you see in post-renal azotemia?	Early phase is similar to pre-renal (BUN/Cr.>15-20) but later is similar to renal azotemia (BUN/Cr.<10)
What are the main features of renal azotemia?	BUN/Cr. <10, Urinary Na>40, Uosm.<350
What are the causes of toxin-	Aminoglycosides, chemotherapy

induced renal insufficiency?	(Cisplatin), contrast dye and amphotericin; they all show muddy brown granular cast
What do you have to order when evaluating contrast induced renal failure?	Mg level
What are the causes of acute interstitial nephritis (AIN)?	Penicillin, phenytoin, cyclosporine, allopurinol, quinidine, quinolones, rifampin
What tests do you order for AIN?	U/A, staining WBC with Wright's or Hansel's technique
What are the differential diagnoses for post exercise dark urine?	Post exercise hematuria and myoglobinuria (can be due to rhabdomyolysis or march trauma to RBC)
What are the causes of rhabdomyolysis?	SICK SA: seizure, immobilization, crush injuries, hypokalemia, statins and alcohol
How do you treat hyperkalemia?	Insulin plus glucose, calcium gluconate
How do you diagnose rhabdomyolysis?	U/A shows myoglobinuria and no cells; CPK and potassium are increased; Ca and bicarbonate are decreased (maybe effect of phosphate on Ca)
What is the treatment of rhabdomyolysis?	Fluids, diuresis and alkalinization of urine by bicarbonate
What is the most important test in myoglobinuria?	EKG to show hyperkalemia
What are the causes of oxaluria?	Antifreeze (ethylene glycol);

	ethanol or fomepizole; immediate dialysis if severe
How do you treat uric aciduria?	Allopurinol and hydration
How do you prevent contrast induced renal failure?	Hydration with normal saline, bicarbonate and N acetylecysteine
What is the mechanism of NSAIDS and kidney damage?	Direct toxicity, allergic interstitial nephritis, vasoconstriction of renal afferent due to PG blockage and nephritic syndrome
What are the main features of glomerulonephritis?	Edema, RBC and RBC casts in urine, >2 g protein in the urine and it may go to nephrotic syndrome
What is the treatment of Goodpasture's syndrome?	Plasmapheresis
What do you see in renal biopsy of Goodpasture's syndrome?	Linear immunofluorescence of basement membrane
What disease is often misdiagnosed with Wegener's granulomatosis?	Pneumonia
What is the best initial test for polyarteritis nodosa (PAN)?	ESR, CRP
What is the most accurate test of PAN?	Biopsy, but angiography showing beading can replace biopsy
What is the most common cause of painless recurrent hematuria plus	IgA nephropathy should be ruled out with biopsy

nephritic syndrome?

What is the treatment of IgA nephropathy (Berger's disease)?	ACE inhibitors, steroids, fish oil however, there is no specific or proven therapy
What is Henoch-Schonlein purpura?	PJRA: purpura, joint, renal and abdominal involvement
What is the most accurate test for HSP? **How do you treat HSP?**	IgA deposits in renal biopsy No treatment
What are the main features of PSGN?	HTN, edema, RBC in urine, low complement, anti DNase, ASO and antihyaluronidase are positive
What is the treatment of PSGN?	Penicillin and diuretics
What are the main features of cryoglobulinemia?	Joints: arthralgia Skin: purpura Nerve: neuropathy RES: lymphadenopathy, hepatosplenomegaly Association: hepatitis C
What lab tests changes do we see in cryoglobulinemia?	IgM is increased, C4 is decreased, biopsy is the most accurate test
Why is it important to biopsy the kidney in SLE?	It shows the extent of the disease: 1. sclerosis alone needs no treatment; 2. mild disease needs steroids; 3. Severe (proliferative) needs mycophenolate and steroids
Why do we see thrombosis in nephrotic syndrome?	Loss of protein C,S & antithrombin in urine
What are the best initial tests for nephrotic syndrome?	U/A, spot urine protein/creatinine>3.5 (mostly in pediatrics) or 24h urine >3.5 g/day (

	mostly in adults) ; most accurate test is biopsy
What is minimal change disease?	Effacement of podocytes and the most common nephrotic syndrome in children
In what group do you see membranous nephropathy?	Lymphoma and adult cancers
In what group do you see MPGN?	Hepatitis C
In what group do you see FSGS?	Heroin and HIV
In what group do you see mesangial glomerulonephritis?	Unclear
How do you approach mild proteinuria?	1st repeat U/A if positive consider transient proteinuria(fever, CHF, exercise & infection) if negative take morning and afternoon samples; if positive in the morning too, do protein/Cr. Spot and if positive do biopsy
What is orthostatic proteinuria?	Proteinuria in the afternoon and not in the morning
What is the treatment of orthostatic proteinuria?	None
What are the indications of dialysis?	If renal failure is present: hyperkalemia, metabolic acidosis, encephalopathy, pericarditis, fluid overload If no renal failure but drug toxicity is present: Li, aspirin and ethylene glycol
What are the treatments for uremia manifestations?	Hypocalcemia: V.D Hypermagnesemia: decrease intake

	Hyperphosphatemia: calcium citrate Anemia: erythropoietin
What is the effect of renal failure on morphine?	Because of low excretion of active metabolites produced in the liver there is potentiation of its effect
What are the clinical features of hypernatremia?	Confusion, seizure and coma
How do you approach hypernatremia?	Either dehydration (fever, pneumonia and poor intake) or diabetes insipidus (nephrogenic or central)
What are the two electrolyte abnormalities that can cause nephrogenic diabetes insipidus?	Hypercalcemia and hypokalemia can cause nephrogenic DI
What are the lab abnormalities in diabetes insipidus?	Uosm is low, urine volume is high, urine Na is low, water deprivation test is negative (no change in urine osmolality)
How do you differentiate central from nephrogenic diabetes insipidus?	DDAVP is given, if it can decrease urine volume and increase Uosm then it is central diabetes insipidus and the treatment is DDAVP
Classify true hyponatremia?	Hyponatremia with hypervolemia: CHF, cirrhosis, nephrotic syndrome Hyponatremia with hypovolemia: GI loss, skin loss, urinary loss (diuretics), Addison's disease (hypoaldosteronism) Hyponatremia with euvolemia: SIADH, psychogenic polydipsia, hypothyroidism
What does cause	Hyperlipidemia, hyperglycemia,

USMLE STEP 3 IN ONE WEEK

pseudohyponatremia?	hyperproteinemia
What are the causes of SIADH?	SSRI and sulfa drugs, any CNS disorder, any lung disease, cancer
What lab abnormalities do you see in SIADH?	Urine Na is high, Uosm is high, serum osmolality is low, Uric acid is low in blood, BUN, Cr and bicarbonate is normal
What is the treatment for hyponatremia?	Mild: water restriction Moderate to severe: normal saline + loop diuretics; 3% normal saline for severe cases (check Na level frequently)
How quickly Na level should be corrected in hyponatremia?	Not faster than 12 unit in the first 24h if sodium is less than 115-120
What are the causes of hyperkalemia?	Renal failure, diuretics, metabolic acidosis, crush injuries, rhabdomyolysis, seizure, low aldosterone including RTA IV, beta blockers, digoxin, low insulin, ACE inhibitors, ARB
How do you treat hyperkalemia?	Insulin with glucose, Ca gluconate, bicarbonate, beta agonist, Kayexelate, if renal failure present dialysis maybe necessary
What are the EKG changes of hyperkalemia?	Peak T waves, wide QRS
What is pseudohyperkalemia?	RBC in tube stays longer and lysis occur leading to hyperkalemia
What are the causes of	BRAVE DAD: Barrter's syndrome,

hypokalemia?	RTA, Aldosterone is high, Vomiting, E is nothing, Diuretics, Amphotericin, Dietary intake is decreased
What EKG changes do you see in hypokalemia?	U wave (Purkinje fiber repolarization)
What are the causes of hypermagnesemia?	Renal failure, antacids, laxatives and iatrogenic
How do you treat hypermagnesemia?	Dietary restriction, saline infusion plus diuresis, dialysis (occasionally) and calcium
What are the main causes of hypomagnesemia?	Decreased absorption: malabsorption, malnutrition & alcoholism Increase renal loss: diuretics, PTH, hypercalcemia, aldosterone Drugs: gentamicin and Cisplatin
What is the treatment of hypomagnesemia?	MgSO4 for acute, Mg oxide for chronic
What are the causes of metabolic acidosis with increased anion gap?	Lactic acidosis, DKA, uremia, aspirin, INH, methanol, ethylene glycol
What are the causes of normal AG metabolic acidosis?	Diarrhea, RTA & hyperalimentation
What are the two main causes of metabolic acidosis+ hypokalemia + hyperchloremia?	Diarrhea is the most common cause otherwise RTA
What is RTA type I?	Can't acidify urine (distal tubule), so they get stones, can't excrete hydrogen ion so treat with bicarbonate

What is RTA type II?	Can't reabsorb HCO3 (proximal tubule); initially urine pH goes up then bicarbonate is lost and pH goes down. Acidemia increases bone resorption and ostomalacia is seen
How do you treat RTA type II?	Treat with diuretics to cause contraction alkalosis (HCO3 is reabsorbed better when less urine is formed)
What is RTA type IV and its most common cause?	Hypoaldosteronism & diabetes; diabetes is causing low sensitivity to aldosterone. treat with fludrocortisone
How do you differentiate between RTA and diarrhea?	Urinary anion gap= Na – Cl; if negative it means Cl is excreted i.e. acid is excreted (NH4Cl). In diarrhea UAG is negative
What are the causes of metabolic alkalosis?	Loss of hydrogen ion from GI (vomiting or NG tube); hyperaldosteronsism (primary or secondary), hypokalemia, Bartter's syndrome, milk alkali syndrome
What are the main features of polycystic kidney disease?	Hematuria, stones and infection; cyst in the brain (aneurysm), cyst in the heart (MV prolapse), cyst in the liver, cyst in the colon (diverticulosis)

What is the most common cause of death in polycystic kidney disease?	ESRD
What is the management of ureteral stones?	If less than 10 mm manage conservatively with hydration and pain control
What is the treatment of stress incontinence?	Kegel exercise, estrogen cream
What is the treatment of urge incontinence?	Behavior therapy, anticholinergics: oxybutynin, tolterodine, trospium, darifenacin, solfenacin
What is the next step if blood pressure is high once?	Repeat in 1-2 weeks
What are the routine tests for HTN?	EKG, U/A, eye and cardiac examination
What is the most effective lifestyle modification?	Weight loss. Other modifications are exercise, low Na and DASH diet
How long do we need for lifestyle modification to show its effect?	3-6 months
What is the first line of treatment in HTN?	In African Americans still it is thiazides otherwise any of thiazides, ACEI, CCB, ARB can be first line unless pt. has BPH (alpha blocker)
How do you treat HTN is one medication isn't enough?	ACEI and CCB given together
What is the next step if 2 medications against HTN don't work?	Add a third drug and investigate for secondary HTN. Also if age is >60 or <30 or there is any specific findings investigate for secondary HTN

What is the most common cause of secondary hypertension in less than 18?	Renal disease (also aortic coarctation must be ruled out)
What are specific findings for renovascular hypertension?	Abdominal bruit plus hypokalemia
What is the best initial test for renal artery stenosis?	Ultrasound and Doppler; if kidney is small do MRA/nuclear scan; if positive findings do angioplasty and stenting
What is the most accurate test in renal artery stenosis?	Angiography
What are the most common cause of secondary hypertension in a young woman between 20-40?	Thyroid diseases, renal diseases and fibromuscular dysplasia
What is the most common cause of secocndary hypertension in middle aged people?	Aldostronism, thyroid diseases, Cushing's, obstructive sleep apnea and pheochromocytoma

Infectious & Immune Diseases

What is the definition of fever of unkown origin?	3 weeks of fever and no diagnosis after basic evaluation. Most common cause is idiopathic then connective tissue, infectious and malignacy
What is the first thing in history of fever in a pt. with travel history?	How many days after he arrived fever developed since it shows the incubation period
What oral or IV antibiotics are effective for methicillin sensitive Staphylococcus aureus?	**Oral is Dicloxacillin/ cephalexin; IV is Dicloxacillin or cefazolin**
What do you use for MRSA minor infection?	Bactrim or clindamycin
What do you use for MRSA severe infection?	VLDT: vancomycin, linezolid, daptomycin, tigecycline
What is the antibiotic of choice in penicillin allergy (not only rash) and severe infection?	VLD but if anaphylaxis use macrolide or clindamycin
What is the antibiotic of choice in penicillin allergy (not only rash) and minor infection?	Macrolides or Bactrim or clindamycin
What is the antibiotic of choice in Streptococcal infection?	All anti Staph. antibiotics including penicillin, ampicillin and amoxicillin
What are the main G-	SPECEM: Serratia, Pseudomona, E coli,

bacteria?	Citrobacter, Enterobacter, Morganella
What kind of cephalosporins do work against G- bacteria?	Cefepime (good choice for neutopenics), ceftazidime
What penicillins are good against G- bacteria?	Piperacillin, ticarcillin
What monobactam is good against G- bacteria?	Aztronem
What quinolones are good against G- bacteria?	Ciprofloxacin, moxifloxacin, levofloxacin
What aminoglycosides are used against G-?	TAG: tobramycin, amikacin, gentamicin
What carbapenems are used against G-?	Imipenem, meropenem, ertapenem
Which carbapenem doesn't work against Pseudomona?	Ertapenem
What antibiotics have excellent coverage for pneumococcal infection?	Levofloxacin, moxifloxacin
How do aminoglycosides act synergistically with beta lactams against G+?	Beta lactam breaks the cell wall and aminoglycoside destroy the ribososmes
What is the carbapenem coverage?	Anaerobes, Staph, Streptococcus, Pseudomona (except ertapenem)
What is tigecycline coverage?	MRSA and G-

What antibiotics have good coverage for GI anaerobes?	Metronidazole, carbapenem, piperacillin, ticarcillin, cefoxitin, cefotetan
What do you use for respiratory anaerobes?	Clindamycin
What antibiotics don't have anaerobe coverage?	Aminoglycosides, quinolones, oxacillin/nafcillin, aztronem and most cephalosporins (except for cefoxitin & cefotetan)
What is effective against cytomegalovirus?	Ganciclovir, foscarnet
What is the toxicity of ganciclovir?	Neutropenia and BM suppression
What is the toxicity of foscarnet?	Renal toxicity
What is effective against both influenza A and B?	Oseltamivir, zanamivir
What do you use against hepatitis C?	Ribavirin and alpha interferon
What is the treatment of respiratory syncytial virus?	Ribavirin
What is the treatment for chronic hepatitis B?	ALITE: Adefovir, Lamivudine, Interferon, Telbivudine, Entecavir
What is the treatment for Candidiasis?	Fluconazole
What is the treatment for Aspergillosis?	Voriconazole

What is the best antifungal for neutropenic fever?	Caspofungin, micafungin, anidulafungin
What are the advantages of echinocandines?	No significant toxicity
What are the disadvantages of echinocandines?	No Cryptococcus coverage
What are the side effects of amphotericin?	Renal toxicity, hypokalemia, metabolic acidosis, fever, chill, shake
What is the best initial test for osteomyelitis?	X-ray first then MRI
Is there any association between osteomyelitis and fracture?	Unless history of open fracture, none.
What is the first sign of osteomyelitis on X-ray?	Periosteal elevation
Is MRI superior to bone scan in osteomyelitis?	Yes. Bone scan can't differentiate between soft tissue infection and osteomyelitis
What is the best marker for osteomyelitis treatment follow-up?	If after 4-6 weeks ESR is still high further treatment and possible surgery is needed
How do you treat G+ osteomyelitis?	IV oxacillin or nafcillin; if MRSA use vancomycin/linezolid/daptomycin
What is the G- osteomyelitis treatment?	Oral antibiotics against Salmonella or Pseudomona
What is the treatment for otitis externa (cellulitis)?	Polymyxin/neomycin/ofloxacin + hydrocortisone, acetic acid and water for ear

USMLE STEP 3 IN ONE WEEK

How do you treat malignant otitis externa ?	Surgery and anti-Pseudomona penicillins such as piperacillin or ticarcillin. Alternatively you can use carbapenem, cefepime
How do you diagnose otitis media?	Clinically by lack of movement of tympanic membrane
What do you do if the best initial treatment of otitis media isn't working? How long do you wait?	Wait for 3 days and if there is no response then use amoxicillin + clavulonate or cefuroxime or ceftibuten, cefprozil, cefdinir
What is the next step if rapid Strep test is negative?	No need to treat
What is the treatment of Strep pharyngitis and penicillin allergy?	Azithromycin or clarithromycin
How do you diagnose influenza?	Ag testing of nasopharyngeal swab
Who gets the flu vaccination?	>50, COPD, CHF, steroids, dialysis, health workers
What is the treatment for impetigo?	Mupirocin (topical) , cephalexin or Dicloxacillin oral; if MRSA used Bactrim or clindamycin of minor and if severe use vancomycin/linezolid/daptomycin
What are different types of hemolysis?	Beta has A,B,C & D subtypes and it means complete hemolysis, alpha is incomplete and gamma means no hemolysis
How do you treat erysipelas	Cephalexin is given before culture and

before culture sample is taken?	when culture comes back
What is the treatment of minor cellulitis?	Oral cephalexin and macrolides if allergy
What is the treatment of severe cellulitis?	IV cefazolin and if allergy use VLD (vancomycin or linezolid or daptomycin)
How do you treat carbuncles and boils?	Similar to cellulitis but surgery may be needed
What is the best initial test in fungal infection?	KOH + acid + heat
How do you treat hair or nail involvement in fungal infection?	Terbinafine (liver function test needed), itraconazole or griseofulvin
What topical antifungals are used if there is no hair or nail involvement?	teraconazole, ecoconazole, clotrimazole, circopirox, miconazole, ketoconazole, nystatin
What is the treatment of urethritis and cervicitis?	Ceftriaxone + azithromycin
How do you diagnose urethritis and cervicitis?	Swab for staining, culture and DNA probe
What infections are seen with terminal complement deficiency?	Recurrent capsular infection e.g. Neisseria
What are the alternatives to urethritis treatment?	Ciprofloxacin + doxycycline
What lab finding is showing the severity of pelvic inflammatory disease?	Leukocytosis

USMLE STEP 3 IN ONE WEEK

What is the definite way to diagnose PID?	Laparoscopy but rarely done
How do you usually diagnose PID?	Cervical culture for gonorrhea and DNA probe for Chlamydia
What is the treatment of PID?	Cefoxitin IV (inpatient) or ceftriaxone IM (outpatient) + doxycycline
What antibiotics are safe in pregnancy?	A PACE: aztronem, penicillins, azithromycin, cephalosporins and erythromycin
How do you treat orchitis?	<35 ceftriaxone + doxycycline; >35 ciprofloxacin
Which genital ulceration has adenopathy?	All of them: syphilis, HSV II, chancroid, LGV
What is the causative agent for lymphogranuloma venerum?	Chlamydia trachomatis
What are the agent and media for chancroid?	H. ducreyi, Muller-Hinton agar or Nairobi medium
How do you treat chancroid?	Ceftriaxone or azithromycin
What is the treatment for lymphogranuloma venerum?	Doxycycline
What is the agent for granuloma inguinale?	Klebsiella granulomatis
How do you treat granuloma inguinale?	Doxycycline or Bactrim
How do you treat scabies &	Permethrin and Lindane respectively

pediculosis?	
What is the treatment for warts?	Mechanical removal (surgery, cryo, podophylin) or imiquimod
What is imiquimod?	An immunostimulant
How do you treat uncomplicated urinary tract infection?	Bactrim for 3 days if < 20% resistance otherwise ciprofloxacin
What is the treatment of complicated urinary tract infection?	Bactrim or ciprofloxacin for 7 days
How do you diagnose UTI in women?	Urinalysis and culture
How do you diagnose UTI in men?	Urinalysis + culture + ultrasonography
When do you treat asymptomatic bacteriuria?	Only in pregnancy
What is the most important finding on urinalysis?	WBC means bacteriuria, leukocyte esterase means granulocytes, nitrites means G- bacteria
How specific are proteins or RBCs in urine?	Not specific at all. It could be infection or glomerulonephritis
What is the treatment of pyelonephritis?	Inpatient: ampicillin+ gentamicin; outpatient: ciprofloxacin
What is the next step if after 5-7 days pyelonephritis doesn't respond to antibiotic therapy?	Evaluate for perinephric abscess

How do you diagnose and treat perinephric abscess?	Biopsy and antibiotics (cipro for G- and oxacillin for Staph)
What does it feel when you examine prostatitis?	Boggy (wet sponge)
How do you treat prostatitis?	Ciprofloxacin for weeks (it is like an abscess)
What is the treatment of infective endocarditis?	Vancomycin + gentamicin for 4-6 weeks
When is surgery indicated in infective endocarditis?	Valve rupture, prosthetic valve, fungal endocarditis, abscess formation, embolic events
When do you need to do colonoscopy in infective endocarditis?	When the agent for infective endocarditis is Strep. bovis
What is the antibiotic of choice for infective endocarditis prophylaxis?	Ampicillin however in the case of infected skin surgery vancomycin or clindamycin
What heart defects do need infective endocarditis prophylaxis?	Cyanotic, valve disease in transplant patients, prosthetic valve and previous infective endocarditis
What procedures do need infective endocarditis prophylaxis?	Dental with bleeding, respiratory tract, infected skinGU/GI surgery
What procedures don't need infective endocarditis prophylaxis?	Filling defects, flexible scopes, OB/GYN, urinary procedures

What cardiac defects don't need prophylaxis?	Valvular diseases, ASD, VSD, Pacemaker & ICD
What is the main difference between Osler's node and Janeway lesions?	Osler's nodes are painful
What are the major Duke's criteria?	2 positive cultures, Echo findings
What are the minor Duke's criteria?	Fever, risk factors, vasculitis, immunological lesions, culture positive
How do you diagnose infective endocarditis by using Duke's criteria?	2 major or 1 major and 3 minor or 5 minor Duke criteria
What are the risk factors for infective endocarditis?	Structural heart disease, IV drug abuser, prosthetic valve, history of infective endocarditis, dental bleeding
What are the signs of vasculitis seen in infective endocarditis?	Janeway lesions, emboli, mycotic aneurysm, conjunctival hemorrhage, splinter hemorrhage
What are the immunological findings in infective endocarditis?	Osler's nodes, Roth's spots in retina, glomerulonephritis
What is the next step in a patient with fever and murmur?	Blood culture and Echo
What do you do if transthoracic Echo is negative in suspected infective endocarditis?	Transesophageal echo
When to do start HIV treatment?	If CD4<350, if symptomatic, if pregnant and in the case of needle stick injury

What is HAART?	LET and RET LET : lamivudine, efavirenz, tenofovir RET: raltegravir, emtricitabine, tenofovir
What are the three groups of antiretroviral medications?	PI (protease inhibitor), NRTI (nucleoside reverse transcriptase inhibitor), NNRTI(non-nucleoside reverse transcriptase inhibitor)
What are the side effects of nucleoside reverse transcriptase inhibitors?	Lactic acidosis (zidovudine, lamivudine, abacavir, emtricitabine)
What are the side effects of PIs (protease inhibitors)?	Hyperglycemia, hyperlipidemia
What is the main side effect of zidovudine?	Anemia
What is the main side effect of indinavir?	Kidney stones
What is the main side effect of didanosine and stavudine?	Pancreatitis and neuropathy
How do you manage needle stick injury, mucosal exposure or unprotected sex in HIV patient?	One month of HAART
What do you do for pregnant and HIV positive?	If under treatment before pregnancy continue with treatment; if CD4<350 treat; if CD4>350 and viral load is low treat during second and third trimester
When do you give	Is CD4<200

prophylaxis for Pneumocystis jiroveci?	
How do you give Pneumocystis prophylaxis?	Bactrim and if allergy to sulfa give atovaquone or dapsone (be careful of G6PD deficiency)
When is the time to give prophylaxis for Mycobacterium avium intracellulare?	CD4<50 then give azithromycin
What is the best initial test for diagnosing PCP?	LDH is increased, dyspnea and dry cough
What is the most accurate test for PCP?	Bronchoalveolar lavage
How do you treat PCP?	Bactrim, pentamidine, atovaquone ; note that dapsone is only for prophylaxis
What are the major adverse effects of pantamidine?	Hypo and hyperglycemia Hypo and hyperkalemia hypocalcemia
When do you give steroids in PCP?	If PO2 <70 or A-a >35
How do you treat toxoplasmosis?	Pyrimethamine + sulfadiazine
What is the best initial test in toxoplasmosis?	Contrast CT
When do you biopsy for suspected toxoplasmosis? When do you see cytomegalovirus infection?	Treat then repeat CT and if the lesion is not getting smaller then brain biopsy is needed CD4<50

How do you treat retinal infection by CMV?	Lifelong valganciclovir unless CD4 goes up with HAART
When do you see Cryptococcus infection?	CD4< 100
How do you diagnose Cryptococcus meningitis?	India ink of CSF is the best initial test then serum CRAG (Cryptococcus Ag)
What is the treatment for Cryptococcus meningitis?	Amphotericin then lifelong fluconazole unless CD4 is up
What is the best initial test for PML (progressive multifocal leukoencephalopathy)?	CT/MRI
What are the main features of PML?	CD4<50, HIV, aphasia, hemiparesis, cortical blindness
What is the treatment of Mycobacterium avium intracellulare (MAI)?	Azithromycin + ethambutol
What are the main features of MAI infection?	Wasting, anemia, alkaline phosphatase, GGTP (gamma glutamyl transpeptidase)
What is the most sensitive test in MAI?	Liver biopsy is more sensitive than bone marrow
How do you treat leptospirosis?	Ceftriaxone or penicillin
What are the 2 types of leptospirosis?	Icteric (Weil's disease) and non-icteric
What are the clinical features of leptospirosis?	Jaundice, history of animal exposure and renal involvement

How do you treat tularemia?	Streptomycin or gentamicin
What is the treatment of cysticercosis?	Albendazole
How do you treat Lyme disease?	Doxycycline, ampicillin if pregnant, ceftriaxone if CNS or cardiac involvement
How do you diagnose Lyme disease?	Serology and PCR or Western blot
What is the treatment of babesiosis?	Quinine, clindamycin
How do you diagnose babesiosis?	Tetrads in RBC seen in smear & PCR
What is Erlichiosis?	G- Infection of monocytes and granulocytes leading to leukopenia
What are the main features of Erlichiosis?	Leukopenia, thrombocytopenia, transaminitis, no rash
How do you treat Erlichiosis?	Doxycycline
What is the treatment for malaria?	Quinine or doxycycline
What is the malaria prophylaxis?	Chloroquine, mefluquine, Malarone (atovaquone + proguanil)
How do you diagnose malaria?	Thin smear
What is the treatment of Nocardiosis?	Bactrim
How do you diagnose	CXR (best initial), culture (most accurate

Nocardiosis (branching filamentous bacteria)?	test)
How do you diagnose actinomycosis?	Staining (G+) & culture
What is the treatment for actinomycosis?	Penicillin
How do you treat acute pulmonary histoplasmosis?	None
How do treat disseminated (pancytopenic) histoplasmosis?	Amphotericin
What are the main clues for diagnosing Histoplasmosis, Coccidioidomycosis, Blastomycosis?	Wet Dry Rural
What are the similarities between histoplasmosis and tuberculosis?	Anything TB does Histoplasma does too
How do you treat Coccidioidomycosis?	Itraconazole
What is the treatment for blastomycosis?	Itraconazole or amphotericin
How do you diagnose blastomycosis?	BBB: broad base budding yeast
What is the treatment for anaphylaxis?	ABCD of CPR and epinephrine SQ (1:1000), steroids and diphenhydramine
What is the main clue in	Minor trauma, ACE inhibitors

angioedema?

How do you diagnose angioedema?	C2 and C4 are decreased
What is the treatment for angioedema? **Is there any place for beta blockers in anaphylaxis management?**	FFP, androgens (danazole) Stop beta blockers before any anaphylaxis treatment
How do you treat allergic rhinitis?	Avoidance, antihistamines, topical steroids, cromolyns, normal saline spray and wash, ipratropium, montelukast, immunotherapy
What antihistamines are used in allergic rhinitis?	Loratadine, fexofenadine, cetirizine
What is the most important finding in primary immunodeficiency?	If lymphatic tissues are present diagnosis is common variable immunodeficiency and if absent it is Bruton's agammaglobulinemia
What is the diagnosis of malabsorption, atopy and recurrent sinopulmonary infection?	IgA deficiency
What kind of transfusion reaction can happen in IgA deficient patients?	Maybe anaphylaxis because IgA is seen as non-self
How do you treat immunodeficiency?	IVIG for Bruton's and CVID, treat infection in IgA deficiency and hyperIgE syndrome
When recurrent Staph. Infections, what Dx should be ruled out?	HyperIgE syndrome

Endocrinology

How do you diagnose diabetes?	Fasting blood glucose is ≥ 126, HbA1C > 6.5, random glucose is 200 and symptoms are present, GTT (2h 75 g) is abnormal
What is the best initial therapy for type II diabetes?	Diet, exercise and weight loss (25% responds)
When is metformin contraindicated?	Renal failure, lactic acidosis and contrast media
What are the most important side effects of sulfonylureas?	Hypoglycemia and SIADH
When is rosiglitazone contraindicated?	CHF
What are the mechanisms of action of acarbose and miglitol?	Alpha glucosidase inhibitors at the brush border which blocks absorption of glucose
What are the important points about nateglinide and repaglinide?	They act similar to sulfonylureas and secret insulin. They are short acting and can cause hypoglycemia
What are –gliflozin medications?	They increase glucose flow in urine
What is the mechanism of action of Exenatide?	GLP-1 analogue which increases insulin secretion and inhibits glucagon
What is the mechanism of action of –gliptins?	DPP4 inhibitor; DPP4 is breaking down GLP-1 normally
How many different types of insulin do we use?	Short-acting: Aspart, Lispro and regular long-acting: glargine (once a day) & NPH (twice a day)

What is the order of duration of action of different types of insulin?	Glargine>NPH>regular>Lispro & Aspart
How do you manage DKA?	IV fluid with NS and if glucose is 200 or less D5W IN insulin and if glucose <200 SQ Phosphate is given if <1 Bicarbonate if pH<6.9
What is the best way to determine severity of DKA and ICU admission?	Bicarbonate level<5 pH<7.1 altered mental status
How do you calculate anion gap?	Na – (Cl + HCO3)
What is the marker of ketosis?	Beta hydroxyl butyrate
What is the main concern about potassium in DKA?	If it is low before treatment it means very low potassium and it is very dangerous
A patient with long term DM has fluctuating glucose level. What is one of the diagnoses that must be ruled out?	Gastroparesis since there is delayed gastric emptying therefore the glucose level fluctuates
What is the work up for gatrsoparesis?	Barium swallow and scope to rule out mechanical obstructions then nuclear scan for gastric emptying
How do you manage gastroparesis?	Low fat small portion frequent meals Erythromycin or metoclopramide Liquid diet or tube feeding as the last measure
What are the differentials for gastroparesis?	DM, trauma and surgery, medications (anticholinergics and opioids), idiopathic
What is the standard calorie intake for tube feeding?	30/kg and add 1 g/kg protein
What is the main danger of refeeding syndrome?	Can cause sudden insulin release which causes hypokalemia, hypomagnesemia, hypophosphatemia

What are the complications of diabetes?	and even death HTN (must be <130 and 80) , eye, kidney and neurological involvement, hyperlipidemia
How do you follow up diabetic patients?	Yearly eye and foot exam; urinalysis for microalbuminuria (if positive start ACE inhibitor)
What is first line in treating HTN in diabetics?	ACE inhibitors
How do you treat diabetic neuropathy?	Gabapentin or pregabalin Increases motilin
What signs are common between hyper and hypothyroidism?	Weakness, myopathy, fatigue and menstrual abnormalities
What are the four causes of hyperthyroidism?	Grave's (treat with radioactive iodine) , silent (no need to treat) subacute (aspirin for treatment), TSH adenoma (surgery for treatment)
What dermopathy is seen in Grave's disease?	Thickening of the skin below the knee (pretibial myxedema)
What nail problem is seen in Grave's?	onycolysis
How do you treat Grave's?	PTU, radioactive iodine, propranolol
What is silent hyperthyroidism?	Leakage from thyroid and everything else is normal
What antibodies are positive in Grave's?	Anti TPO (thyroid peroxidase) , anti TSH receptor

What antibodies are seen in silent hyperthyroidism?	Anti TPO, anti-thyroglobulin
How do you treat thyroid storm?	Iodine (blocks absorption), PTU (blocks production), beta blockers (blocks the effect of thyroid hormones), dexamethasone (decreases conversion of T4 to T3)
What Ab is seen in Hashimoto's disease?	Anti-thyroglobulin Ab
What is the next step in the management of solitary thyroid nodule?	Fine needle aspiration unless TSH is low and there is no risk factors. If thyroid scan shows hot nodule no need to do FNA
What is the most common presentation of hyperparathyroidism?	Ultrasonography and TSH: if TSH is high or normal do FNA otherwise do scan (if cold nodule do FNA)
What is the most common presentation of hyperparathyroidism?	Asymptomatic
What are the main features of refractory secondary hyperparathyroidism?	In chronic renal failure when hypercalcemia happens due to very high PTH and also phosphate is high plus soft tissue calcification
What is the mechanism of hypercalcemia in granulomatous diseases?	Epitheloid cells in granuloma make alpha 1 hydroxylase which makes active form of V.D
How do you workup hypercalcemia?	First check PTH level and if it is high check urinary Ca level. If urine Ca is high hyperparathy. Is the diagnosis and if it is low Familial hypocalciuric hypercalcemia is the diagnosis

	If PTH is normal or low it can be: malignancy, sarcoidosis and other granulomatous diseases, thiazides, V.D intoxication
What are the main clinical features of hyperparathyroidism?	Stones, bones, psychogenic moans, abdominal groans
What is the indication of surgical removal of parathyroid adenoma?	Symptomatic, calcium is markedly elevated in 24h urine, serum calcium >12.5, renal insufficiency
What is euthyroid sick syndrome?	Normal thyroid function except for some lab abnormality mostly low T3
What are the clinical features of hypercalcemia?	Nephrogenic diabetes insipidus: polyuria, polydipsia, confusion, constipation, decrease QT interval, ATN, stones, renal insufficiency
How do you treat hypercalcemia?	Fluid, maybe furosemide, steroids for granulomatous diseases, bisphosphonates, calcitonin (short term)
What malignancies do cause hypercalcemia?	Lungs, head and neck and esophageal SCC Breast, ovarian and endometrial carcinoma Renal and bladder carcinoma
What are the causes of hypocalcemia?	Surgery (iatrogenic), low Mg, low V.D, acute hyperphosphatemia, PTH resistance
What is the mechanism of hypocalcemia caused by hyperphosphatemia?	Phosphate binds calcium and lowers it
What is the mechanism of hypocalcemia caused by	Mg is needed for PTH action

hypomagnesemia?	
What EKG changes do you see in acute hypocalcemia?	Prolonged QT
What tests do you do for diagnosis of Cushing's syndrome?	1. 1 mg dexamethasone if suppressed do nothing 2. If not suppressed do 24h urinary cortisol if negative check false positive causes of 1 mg dexamethasone 3. If 24h cortisol is positive check ACTH if high do high dose of dexamethasone if suppression happens it is Cushing's disease then do MRI. If can't suppress do CT chest to rule out lung carcinoma 4. If ACTH is not high check adrenal gland
What are the causes of false positive 1 mg dexamethasone suppression test?	Depression, alcoholism, stress
What is the workup for adrenal insufficiency?	Check ACTH and cortisol level after cosyntropin stimulation test: if ACTH is high and cortisol stays low even after stimulation it is primary adrenal failure If ACTH is low it is secondary
What are the main clinical features of Addison's disease?	Hypoglycemia, hyponatremia, hyperkalemia, neutropenia (no steroids)
What is the effect of glucocorticoids on WBC and glucose?	Increases both

What is the most accurate tests for Addison's?	ACTH (cosyntropin) stimulation test can't increase cortisol
What is the effect of aldosterone on kidney tubules?	Na/K exchange pump in distal and collecting tubules plus secretion of hydrogen ion in collecting duct intercalated cells
What is the treatment of Addison's?	Fluid and hydrocortisone in acute cases and when stable use prednisone and if BP is still low use fludrocortisone
What are the main features of hyperaldosteronism?	Low renin, metabolic alkalosis, HTN
What is the effect of hypokalemia caused by hyperaldosteronism on kidneys?	Causes nephrogenic diabetes insipidus
What is the one disease that should be ruled out in episodic hypertension?	Pheochromocytoma
What are the best initial tests for pheochromocytoma?	Serum catechol amines, urinary catechol amines, plasma metanephrines, urine MVA
How do you confirm diagnosis of pheochromocytoma?	CT/MRI
How do you diagnose metastatic pheochromocytoma?	MIBG
How do you treat	1st block alpha and then beta

pheochromocytoma?	adrenergics, surgery
Why do you need to block alpha before beta in pheochromocytoma?	Severe HTN can happen if you block beta first, it is because of unopposed alpha effects
What are the three types of congenital adrenal hyperplasia?	21, 11 and 17 hydroxylase deficiency
What tests do you order for 21 hydroxylase deficiency?	17 hydroxy progesterone
What is the difference between 21 and 11	21 deficiency has hypotension and 11 has hypertension
What is the main feature of 17 hydroxylase deficiency?	No virilization
What is the most common pituitary adenoma?	Prolactinoma
Why do we see late presentation in male?	In female amenorrhea happens quickly in male you have to wait for gynecomastia and loss of libido
What is the mechanism of amenorrhea in hyperprolacinoma?	Prolactin inhibits GnRH
What do you do before a workup for prolactinoma?	Rule out pregnancy Exclude durgs like phenothiazines and metoclopramide Rule out hypothyroidism (TRH has positive effect on prolactin) Level must be >200 then other causes of high prolactin are ruled out (nipple stimulation, exercise, stress, chest wall diseases)

What is the most accurate test for prolactinoma?	MRI
How do you treat prolactinoma?	Medical treatment: cabergoline or bromocriptine and if medical treatment fails do surgery
What are the main features of acromegaly?	big head (hat gets smaller), big shoes (shoes get smaller), chin, nose, face and hands get bigger, HTN, cardiomegaly, joint disease (cartilage grows), amenorrhea (high prolactin), diabetes (GH is diabetogenic), colon polyps
How do you diagnose acromegaly?	IGF is the best initial test because it has high half-life; most accurate test is glucose suppression test; MRI is the last test
What if glucose can suppress GH secretion?	Acromegaly is ruled out
How do you treat acromegaly?	SCOPE: Surgery, Cabergoline, Octreotide, Pegvisomant
Why do we have no testosterone in Kleinfelter's?	LG and FSH have no receptors on the testes so they are high but no testosterone
What is the treatment of Kleinfelter's?	Testosterone
What is Kallman's syndrome?	Anosmia and hypogonadism

Oncology

What are the high risk groups for breast carcinoma?	2 first degree 3 first and second degree 1 first degree with bilateral breast carcinoma 1 first degree with ovarian and breast carcinoma Male carcinoma in family
What is the next step if mammogram is abnormal?	Biopsy, if sentinel node is negative no need for axillary node dissection
When do you give adjuvant chemotherapy in breast carcinoma?	If tumor is >1 cm and if axillary involvement is seen
What types of hormone inhibition therapy do we use in breast carcinoma?	SERM (tamoxifen and raloxifen) and aromatase inhibitors (anastrazole, letrozole, exemestane)
What are the side effects of SERM (selective estrogen receptor modulator?	DVT, hot flashes and endometrial hyperplasia (a precancerous lesion)
What is the mechanism of action of SERM?	Partial agonist of estrogen
What are the side effects of aromatase inhibitors?	Osteoporosis
What is the mechanism of action of trastuzumab?	Monoclonal Ab against HER2/Neu Ag in breast cancer. It is used in metastasis

What do you give for preventing breast carcinoma in a patient with multiple 1st degree cancer diagnosis?	Tamoxifen
What is the significance of BRCA?	Breast cancer and ovarian cancer seen in some families
What is the next step in a smoker with solitary lung nodule?	Excisional biopsy especially if >50
What are the cases of non-resectable lung cancer?	Bilateral metastasis, 1-2 cm from carina, pleural effusion, heart/vena cava/aorta involvement
When do you start Pap smear?	Start at 21 after that every 3 years
Who is a candidate for HPV vaccine?	11-26
What is the next step for abnormal Pap smear?	Colposcopy and biopsy
What is abnormal Pap smear?	Low grade or high grade dysplasia
How do you manage high grade dysplasia?	Excision or ablation
What is the next step in ASCUS (atypical squamous cells with undetermined significance)?	HPV testing and if negative repeat in 6 months, if positive colposcopy In young pateints 21-24 repeat Pap smear in one year and if negative repeat again in one year and if negative go back to routine Pap
What is the most common complication of TURP?	Retrograde ejaculation however immediately post op hyponatremia due to flushing solution

USMLE STEP 3 IN ONE WEEK

What is the most important prognostic factor in prostate carcinoma?	Level of differentiation based on Gleason score
How do you treat localized prostate carcinoma?	Surgery plus radiation (external or implanted pellets)
How do you treat metastatic prostate carcinoma?	Block androgens flutamide (testosterone receptor block) and GnRH agonists like goserelin or leuprolide
What is the mechanism of action of finasteride?	5 alpha reductase inhibitor used in BPH and hair loss
What do you use in cord compression due to prostate carcinoma?	GnRH but don't use it in the beginning it can flare up (use flutamide instead)
When do you resect ovarian tumors?	If the tumor is large and spreads throughout the abdomen
When do you biopsy testicular cancer?	Never
What are the testicular cancers?	Germ cell tumors (95%) and non-germ cell tumors; germ cells are divided into seminoma and non-seminoma
What tests are used for testicular cancers?	AFP, LDH, beta hCG, CT for staging; 95 % have 5 year survival rate
How do you treat local testicular cancer?	Radiation
How do you treat widespread testicular cancer?	Chemotherapy which can even treat metastatic diseases

Up to what age Pap smear is done?	65
Who should receive meningococcal vaccine?	At 11 or earlier if they have asplenia or terminal complement deficiency
What age group needs influenza and pneumococcus vaccines?	Influenza for >50 and pneumococcus >65
Who gets screened for osteoporosis?	Women >65
Who needs screening for abdominal aortic aneurysm?	Men >65 who smoke or have smoked in the past

Dermatology

What are the main features of pemphigoid?	Older age usually no oral lesion, deeper blisters, less likely to rupture, immunofluorescence autoantibodies
How do you treat pemphigoid?	Steroids or tetracycline or erythromycin with nicotinamide
What are the main features of pemphigus?	Younger patient (30s or 40s), painful but not pruritic, severe disease, blisters are intraepidermal and break easily, mouth lesion, Nikolsky's sign, Ab against Ag in intercellular space of epidermis, sulfa drugs can precipitated that
What is the treatment of pemphigus?	Steroids, azathioprine, mycophenolate and cyclophosphamide. ACE inhibitors and penicillamine can cause pemphigus
What are the differentials for Nikolsky's sign?	Pemphigus, TEN (toxic epidermal necrolysis) ,SSS (scalded skin syndrome)
What is pemphigus foliaceus?	It is more superficial than pemphigus, no blisters no oral lesions. Diagnosis is biopsy and treatment is steroids
What are the main features of PCT	Blisters on sun exposed areas

(porphyria cutanea tarda?	which don't heal, hyperpigmentation, hypertrichosis of face
What diseases are associated with PCT?	Liver diseases (chronic hepatitis C, hemosiderosis), diabetes, alcoholism, oral contraceptives
How do you diagnose PCT?	Uroporphyrin is up to 5 times more than coproporphyrin
How do you teat PCT?	Avoid alcohol and estrogen, sunscreen protection, phlebotomy & deferoxamine, chloroquine
What is the duration of urticaria?	Usually less than 24h. If episodes lasts more than 6 weeks it is chronic
What drugs usually cause urticarial?	NSAIDS including aspirin, penicillin, codeine, morphine, phenytoin, quinolones
What are the causes of chronic urticaria?	Cold, vibration, pressure on skin
How do you treat urticaria?	If acute use H1 blocker and if it is more severe add H2 blocker and oral steroids. If chronic and not imporved by 2nd generation H1 blockers in 2 weeks add H1 first generation
When is desensitization indicated?	When you can't avoid the triggering factor e.g. a farmer with bee sting urticarial
What is considered as morbiliform rash?	Generalized maculopapular rash which is blanched with pressure; seen with drug allergy even if you have stopped the

	drug earlier (sulfa, penicillin, allopurinol, phenytoin)
What is the treatment of morbiliform rash due to drug hypersensitivity?	Usually antihistamines are enough but rarely steroids are given
What is erythema multiform?	Target lesions on palms and soles without mucosal involvement
What are the causes of erythema multiform?	Herpes simplex, mycoplasma, drugs: SPAN (sulfa, penicillin, antiepileptics, NSAIDS)
How do you treat erythema multiform?	Treat underlying disease and use antihistamines
What are the main features of Steven Johnson's syndrome?	Mucosal involvement is the main feature and it can be very extensive in respiratory system. SPAN can cause that (sulfa, penicillin, antiepileptics, NSAIDS
How do you treat Steven Johnson's syndrome?	Mechanical ventilation if respiratory involvement; admit to burn unit, supportive therapy, no proven benefit with the use of steroids, IVIG, cyclosporine, thalidomide
What is toxic epidermal necrolysis (TEN)?	The most serious form of drug hypersensitivity with more than 70% of skin involved, up to 50 % mortality, most common cause of death is sepsis ; no antibiotic prophylaxis or steroids is recommended
How do you teat fixed drug reaction?	Topical steroids

USMLE STEP 3 IN ONE WEEK

What are the differentials for erythema nodosum?	Sarcoidosis, TB, IBD, Histoplasmosis, Coccidioidomycosis, hepatitis, Yersinia and other enteric infection, Steptococcal infection, syphilis, pregnancy
What is the most accurate test for fungal infection?	Culture but it takes minimum 6 weeks
How do you treat fungal hair or nail infection?	Terbinafine for 6 weeks for fingernail, 12 weeks for toenail, itraconazole
What is the main side effect of terbinafine?	Hepatotoxicity
What side effects ketoconazole has? How do you treat bacterial skin infection if there is penicillin allergy?	Hepatotoxicity, gynecomastia Macrolide or quinolones and if severe MRSA infection use IV vancomycin
When do you use ciprofloxacin in skin infection?	Never
What is the most common cause of impetigo?	Staphylococcus (not Strep. anymore)
How do you treat erysipelas?	Start with broad spectrum antibiotics and if the result of culture shows Strep. use penicillin
What is the treatment of cellulitis?	IV oxacillin/nafcillin or cefazolin (aspiration not very sensitive therefore, use empiric therapy)
What bacteria is causing folliculitis in whirlpool?	Pseudomona, also it causes pneumonia in cystic fibrosis

USMLE STEP 3 IN ONE WEEK

How do you treat carbuncles and furuncles?	Dicloxacillin
Where is the infection in erysipelas, cellulitis and necrotizing fasciitis?	Dermis, subcutaneous tissue and fascia respectively
What are the necrotizing fasciitis manifestations?	Fever, pain out of proportion, crepitation, bullae, history of diabetes, increased CRP, air in the tissue on CT/MRI/X-ray
What is the best initial step in the management of necrotizing fasciitis?	Surgery and antibiotics (ampicillin plus sulbactam/ ticarcillin + clavulunate/ piperacillin + tazobactum)
What is the empirical treatment in necrotizing fasciitis?	PVC (Vanco + Clinda + piperacillin tazobactam) IVC (imipenem + vanco + clinda)
How do you treat necrotizing fasciitis if Strep. pyogen is the cause?	Penicillin plus clindamycin
What is the mortality rate of necrotizing fasciitis?	Up to 90% if untreated and up to 40% if treated
What is paronychia and how do you treat it?	Infection of the skin surrounding the nail; treatment is local incision and anti-Staphylococcus antibiotics
What is the main feature of herpes infection of genitals?	Multiple painful vesicles
What is the significance of Tzanck smear?	It isn't specific and shows only Herpes family
When is Tzanck smear the best initial test?	When there is ulceration and the diagnosis isn't clear

What is the most accurate test for herpes infection?	Culture (not serology)
How effective is topical acyclovir in herpes infection?	Very little effect
How effective is topical penciclovir in herpes infection?	There is some efficacy if used every 2h
What is the best treatment for herpes if it is resistant to acyclovir/famciclovir/valecyclovir?	Foscarnet
What are the complications of varicella?	PHD: pneumonia, hepatitis, dissemination)
How do you manage Varicella zoster?	Tzanck smear and culture rarely needed; treat with steroids, acyclovir, gabapentin, tricyclic antidepressant, capsaicin, IgG within 4 days if non-immune
How long does it take to see the effect of imiquimod for warts?	It takes several weeks to work.
What is the sensitivity of VDRL & RPR in secondary syphilis?	100% but in primary is 75% and dark field microscopy is recommended
When can you see neurosyphilis?	It can happen during secondary (meningitis, ocular) or tertiary syphilis (tabes, dementia
What is the treatment for primary or secondary syphilis?	Single injection of benzathine penicillin or 2 weeks of tetracycline

USMLE STEP 3 IN ONE WEEK

What is Norwegian scabies?	Severe crusting form of scabies in HIV or immune deficiency
How do you diagnose scabies?	Use mineral oil on the burrows and scrape out Sarcoptes scabies
How do you treat Norwegian scabies?	Permethrin topically or Ivermectin orally
When do you give lindane for scabies?	It is neurotoxic (seizure and death) and must be used if other fails
What is the best way to diagnose pedicuclosis?	Inspect the hair
How do you treat pediculosis?	Permethrin or over the counter pyrethrins
What is the usual size of target lesion rash in Lyme's disease?	5 cm; it appears usually 7-10 days after tick bite
Between the rash and serology which is more important in Lyme's diagnosis?	Rash is more important and if seen start with doxycycline/ampicillin/cefuroxime
What are the main features of toxic shock syndrome?	Fever & hypotension, vomiting, skin and mucosa desquamation, CNS dysfunction, Cr.is high, CPK and LFT are increased, platelets decreased
How do you treat TSS?	Anti-staph. antibiotics, fluids and vasopressors
What are the main features of staphylococcal scalded syndrome?	Normal blood pressure, no liver/kidney/CNS damage is seen; it isn't a full thickness skin disease, admit to burn unit

How do you treat anthrax?	Ciprofloxacin or doxycycline; 20% mortality if untreated
How do you differentiate benign from malignant pigmented skin lesion?	ABCDE: asymmetry, border, color, diameter, elevation
What are the types of melanoma?	Superficial spreading (most common), lentigo maligna (sun exposed old people), acral lentiginous (African Americans, extremities), nodular (worst)
How do you treat melanoma?	Excision and interferon
What is keratosis?	Increased stratum corneum
What are the two main diseases with keratosis?	Actinic and seborrheic; actinic is precancerous, sun exposed areas; seborrheic is stuck-on appearance, greasy hyperpigmented on shoulder, face, chest and back
How do you treat senile keratosis?	5FU, cryo, imiquimod, retinoic acid derivatives, curettage
What is Moh's microsurgery?	Instant frozen section for the treatment of basal cell carcinoma which has the greatest cure rate
What is the cause of Kaposi's sarcoma?	HSV8
How do you treat Kaposi's?	Antiretroviral treatment and if it doesn't work use liposomal Adriamycin plus vinblastine
What are the main treatment options	1st Eucerin, Lubriderm,

for psoriasis?	aquaphor, Vaseline, mineral oil. 2nd Salicylates 3rd Steroids if localized 4th Coal tar if severe 5th Topical V.A and V.D (tazarotane & calcipotriene) 6th If >30% involved UV therapy is the fastest 7th If widespread use methotrexate 8th TNF inhibitors: infliximab, etanercept, efalizumab
How do you prevent atopic dermatitis?	No hot water, no drying soap, use emollients and cotton clothes
What is the treatment of atopic dermatitis?	Topical steroids, antihistamines, phototherapy, coal tars, antibiotics against Staph. (impetigo superimposed), topical immunosuppressant (tacrolimus) doxepin for pruritus, don't scratch the rash
What is seborrheic dermatitis?	Oversecretion of sebum and hypersensitivity to fungus (Pityrisporum ovale)
How do you treat seborrheic dermatitis?	Hydrocortisone + ketoconazole/selenium sulfide or zinc pyrithione shampoo
What are the main signs of seborrheic dermatitis?	Dandruff, scaly greasy flaky skin on a red base
What is the definite diagnosis of contact dermatitis?	Patch test
What is the pattern in Pityriasis rosea?	Herald patch and then Christmas tree pattern

	Use low dose UV light for treatment
How do you treat acne step by step?	1st benzyl hydroxide, then add retinoic in the evening, then topical erythromycin/clindamycin finally use oral isotretinoin for nodular cystic ones
What is the treatment of acne rosacea?	Metronidazole cream

Surgery

What are the stages of decubitus ulcer?	I: nonblanching erythema II: shallow ulcer III: deep ulcer IV: extensive destruction of muscle and bone
When do you see subphrenic abscess?	**Usually 2-3 weeks after abdominal surgery**
What is the most common indication for airway intubation?	**Unconsciousness**
What is the most common form of intubation?	Endotracheal
When do you use flexible bronchoscope?	Spinal injury
What do you do if flexible bronchoscope isn't available in spinal injury?	Orotracheal with manual neck stabilization
When do you use cricothyrotomy or percutaneous tracheostomy?	Extensive facial trauma and bleeding
What do you do if pulse oximetry is <90%?	Increased flow rate, ABG, find out the cause of hypoxia
What are the 3 main causes of circulatory collapse?	Hypovolemia, tension pneumothorax and temponade

How do you differentiate tension pneumothorax from temponade?	Tension pneumothorax: No breath sounds on one side, trachea shifted to other side, hyperresonance Temponade: enlarged heart on X-ray, pulsus paradoxus, electrical alternans on EKG
How do you treat tension pneumothorax?	1st large bore needle then chest tube
What is the treatment for temponade?	Pericardiocentesis or window
What test is very helpful in blunt cardiac injury?	ECG
What is the first step in abdominal trauma with open bleeding?	Direct pressure, fluid, prepare for operation: NPO, IV saline, antibiotics, Foley, type and screen
When do you give intraosseous fluid?	<6 year old or in CPR of adults without good access to veins
What are the causes of vasomotor shock?	Drugs, spinal anesthesia, allergens
How do you treat vasomotor shock?	Vasoconstrictors and fluid
What is the management of comminuted or depressed skull fracture?	Operate even if asymptomatic
What do you need to give before open skull fracture?	Tetanus toxoid along with antibiotics

USMLE STEP 3 IN ONE WEEK

What are the main features of basilar skull fracture?
Otorrhea, rhinorrhea, Battle sign, raccoon eye sign, CN palsy VI, VII, VIII; diagnosis is made by CT of head and neck

How do you treat basilar skull fractures?
Steroids for facial nerve palsy, no antibiotics needed for CSF leakage

When is surgery indicated in subdural hematoma?
Midline shift, lateralizing signs

How do you treat subdural hematoma conservatively?
Steroids

What are the signs of subdural hematoma?
Headache, drowsiness, undulating LOC, confusion, personality changes, memory loss

What are the features of diffuse axonal injury?
Deep coma, bad prognosis, mechanism is acceleration deceleration, treat increased ICP

How do you treat increased intracranial pressure?
Head elevation, hyperventilation, avoid fluid overload, mannitol, furosemide, sedation, hypothermia

What are the important clues to increased ICP?
Gradual dilation of one eye, decreasing responsiveness to light

What do you see on CT of the head if ICP is increased?
Midline shift and dilated ventricles

What happens if you do LP in increased ICP?
Death

What cases of acute abdomen are treated medically?
Pancreatitis, diverticulitis, cholangitis, urinary stones and pyelonephritis, MI, GERD, hepatitis, lower lobe pneumonia, pulmonary emboli, ruptured ovarian cyst,

	sickle cell anemia, porphyria, DKA, adrenal insufficiency
What cases of acute abdomen are treated surgically?	Perforation, peritonitis, acute intestinal ischemia, AAA, pain + signs of sepsis, appendicitis
What are the signs of acute GI perforation?	Acute sudden severe constant generalized pain
What are the causes of acute GI perforation?	Peptic ulcer disease, diverticulitis, IBD, esophageal rupture
How do you diagnose GI perforations?	Supine and erect abdominal X-ray
What is the management of GI perforations?	NPO, fluid, antibiotics (cefotetan/cefoxitin or metronidazole + gentamicin), emergent surgery
How do you diagnose esophageal perforations?	Gastrograffin swallow and surgery
What are the signs of obstruction?	No gas passing, vomiting, colicky pain, patient constantly is moving
What are the differentials of intestinal obstruction?	Volvulus, large bowel obstruction (usually due to cancer), intussusception, adhesions (small bowel obstruction), hernias
What are the important clues in the history of a patient suspected of intestinal obstruction?	Prior surgery (adhesion), weight loss or anemia (cancer), recurrent pain (diverticulitis), hernia (incarceration), sudden pain (volvulus)
How do you diagnose	CBC, lactate, supine (absence of air in the

intestinal obstruction?	rectum) and erect (multiple dilated loops and bird beak sign) X-ray
What is the general treatment of intestinal obstruction?	NGT, NPO, Normal saline, gastrograffin if contrast studies needed, surgery is usually the course of action
How do you treat volvulus?	Proctosigmoidoscopy and if it is recurrent resection
What is the treatment for hernia?	Elective surgery unless incarcerated/signs of sepsis or peritonitis which needs emergent surgery
How do you treat diverticulitis?	If no signs of peritoneal irritation treat as an outpatient with antibiotics; if local peritonitis admit (NPO, IV antibiotics and fluid); if recurrent attack elective surgery; if signs of generalized peritonitis emergent surgery
What are the three different forms of pancreatitis?	Edematous Hemorrhagic Suppurative
What are the late complications of pancreatitis?	Pseudocyst, chronic pancreatitis
How do you manage pancreatic pseudocysts?	<6 cm and <6 weeks needs observation; > 6 cm and >6 weeks needs percutaneous drainage under CT or endoscopic drainage
What is pancreatic abscess?	Usually 10 days after pancreatitis there is persistent fever and leukocytosis; treatment is surgical drainage
What lab findings are signs of severe pancreatitis?	Glucose is high, leukocytes are high, BUN is high, hematocrit is high, calcium is low

How do you diagnose appendicitis?	Clinical ; CT and ultrasonography helps
What kind of antibiotics is needed for surgical treatment of appendicitis?	None
What are the indications of surgery in ulcerative colitis?	Toxic megacolon, >20 years duration; multiple hospitalization, high dose of steroid or immunosuppressive needed
How do you diagnose toxic megacolon?	Gas in the wall of colon on X-ray + massively distended colon; toxic signs
How do you manage toxic megacolon?	NPO & NGT for bowel rest IV fluid & electrolytes Antibiotics Steroids unless C. diff is suspected etiology Hold antiperistaltis
How do you diagnose ischemic colitis?	Pain out of proportion to physical exam in an old person with PMH of MI, atrial fibrillation + lactic acidosis and signs of sepsis
What is the treatment of ischemic colitis?	Surgery (embolectomy or revascularization) or angiography (vasodilation and thrombolysis)
How do you diagnose intra-abdominal abscess?	CT with contrast
What are the causes of surgical jaundice?	Obstructive jaundice: 1. Stone 2. Tumor
What is the next step if bile ducts dilated on sonography and gallbladder isn't?	ERCP confirms diagnosis and can treat it
What is the mechanism of	Excess amount of secondary bile salts in

diarrhea in post cholecystectomy patients? What is the surgical treatment of gallstones?	the lumen stimulates colonic mucosa however is seen in only 10% Spincterotomy or cholecystectomy
What are the three tumors causing surgical jaundice?	Carcinoma of head of pancreas Carcinoma of ampulla of Vater Collangiocarcinoma of common bile duct
How do you diagnose the tumors causing jaundice?	Do CT if negative do ERCT and if CT positive perform percutaneous biopsy
What is the treatment for different forms of gallstone presentations?	1. If asymptomatic no treatment unless >3 cm or calcified gallbladder 2. Biliary colic: elective surgery 3. Cholecystitis : elective surgery in 6-12 weeks 4. Cholecystitis with peritonitis: emergent surgery
How do you diagnose acute ascending cholangitis?	Triad of pain, jaundice and fever with very high alkaline phosphatase
What is the treatment of ascending cholangitis?	Antibiotics, IV fluid, decompression of common bile duct with ERCP/PTC Surgery (rarely done), eventually cholecystectomy
What medications can continue during operation?	Betablockers, statins, alpha 2 agonists and CCB Diuretics hold the day of surgery, ACEI only for CHF otherwise hold the night before
What is the management of there is preoperative risk of CHF?	Start ACE inhibitors, beta blockers and diuretics
When do you stop SERM medication before surgery?	4 weeks before because of risk of DVT with them

What is the next step if symptoms of CHF got worse in the past 1-2 years?	Cardiac workup is necessary
When do you have almost 100% mortality in liver diseases if you operate?	If 4 signs of liver disease present: PT >16, albumin<3, bilirubin>2, encephalopathy; if 3 signs are present 85% mortality and if 2 signs are present 40% mortality
What happens if FEV1<1.5 and you operate?	High risk of post-op pneumonia
Can you operate if EF<35%?	No, except for cardiac surgery
What do you do for a patient with CHF before surgery?	ACE inhibitors, beta blockers and diuretics before surgery
If a patient has recent MI can you operate?	No surgery for 6 months
What is the management of severe progressive angina before operation?	Cardiac catheterization
What should the smoker do before operation?	Quit smoking at least 8 weeks before surgery; FEV1<1.5 and high PCO2 show ventilation compromise
When do you give nutritional support 5-10 days before surgery?	When there is a nutritional risk: loss of 20% body weight in recent months, albumin<3, anergy to skin testing, transferrin <200
Can a patient with diabetic coma have surgery?	Absolutely contraindicated

USMLE STEP 3 IN ONE WEEK

What are the risk factors for noncardiac surgery?	1. Age>75 2. Cardiac status: JVD, gallop, significant aortic stenosis, >4 PVC/minute, arrhythmias other than sinus or PAC) 3. General medical condition 4. Type of surgery
What general medical conditions are important in assessing surgery risk for noncardiac surgery?	PO2<60, PCO2>50, K<3, BUN>50, Cr.>3, bed bound patients, elevated AST, chronic liver disease
What kinds of operations are carrying more risks?	Emergent> intraperitoneal/intrathoracic
How patient risk factors affect most ambulatory surgeries?	In general ambulatory surgeries can be done without preop. evaluation
What are the differentials for post-op fever?	1st day in Wind (atelectasis), 3rd day is Water (UTI), 5th day is Walk (thrombophlebitis), 7th day is Wound (wound infection and pulmonary), 10-14 days after deep abscesses
What are the differentials if the post-op patient is disoriented?	Hypoxia (ABG), hyponatremia, hyperglycemia, hypernatremia, uremia, high ammonium, delirium tremens
What is the management of post-op leakage of GI contents to the outside?	Observe because most of them heal. A fecal fistula in a febrile patient with systemic signs is an indication of drainage with a diverting colostomy.
When is TPN first choice?	Almost never, always start nutrition via the gut if possible
Sudden onset of hyperglycemia in a patient	Rule out sepsis, steroids, fast flow of TPN

with TPN?	
How do you treat malignant hyperthermia?	100% O2, dantrolene, cooling blankets, correct acidosis, watch for myoglobinuria
How do you treat post-op bacteremia (high fever)?	Three times blood culture and empiric antibiotic therapy
What treatment is contraindicated in post-up MI?	Don't give thrombolytics
How do you manage 1st post-op day fever?	Spirometry
How do you manage 3rd post-up day fever?	Urinalysis and culture
How do you manage 5th post-up day fever?	Doppler the leg and pelvic veins & start anticoagulation
How do you manage post-up deep abscesses?	CT for diagnosis and treatment via percutaneous drainage
How do you diagnose post-up pulmonary embolism?	CT angiogram, treat with anticoagulation and if recurs IVC filter
How do you manage post-up aspirations?	Lavage and remove gastric contents, bronchodilators and ventilator support
What is the diagnosis if in the OR suddenly BP goes down steadily, CVP is increasing and the patient has positive pressure ventilation?	Tension pneumothorax
What if the post-op patient has tachycardia, hyperthermia, tremor, high blood pressure and altered mental status?	Delirium tremens is the diagnosis and you should treat with benzodiazepines; also watch for seizures and rhabdomyolysis

USMLE STEP 3 IN ONE WEEK

What is the workup for VACTER?

In physical exam look for anus; do X-ray for vertebrae, Echo for cardiac and ultrasonography for renal anomalies

How do you treat tracheoesophageal fistula?

Surgery and if more time is needed for surgery do gastrostomy

How do you treat imperforated anus?

If there is vaginal or perineal fistula present delay surgery otherwise perform colostomy for high rectal pouches

What is the treatment for congenital diaphragmatic hernia?

Intubation and low pressure ventilation, sedation, NG suction, surgery after a few days

What is omphalocele?

Cord goes to the defect

What is gastroschisis?

Cord is to the lateral side of the defect and loops of intestine are seen naked

How do you treat omphalocele or gastroschisis?

Surgery: small defects are closed, large defects need silastic material (Silo) to protect the bowel and manual replacement of the bowel daily for 1 week
life

Which is more dangerous: malrotation, duodenal atresia or annular pancreas?

Malrotation is more dangerous because of twisted loops of intestine

How do you treat bladder extrophy?

Immediate surgery in the 1st or 2nd of

What is the diagnosis if you see multiple air fluid level in a newborn?

Intestinal atresia

USMLE STEP 3 IN ONE WEEK

What surgical diseases are seen in the first 2 months of life?	Hirschprung's, necrotizing enterocolitis, meconium ileus, pyloric stenosis, biliary atresia
What is the diagnosis of a premature baby with rapidly decreasing platelets, signs of sepsis, feeding problems and abdominal distention?	Necrotizing enterocolitis; treat with: stop feeding, antibiotics, IV fluid, surgery if necrosis or perforation (portal vein gas, gas in the abdominal or bowel wall, abdominal wall erythema)
What is the diagnosis of a newborn with bilious vomiting, feeding intolerance, family history of cystic fibrosis and X-ray shows ground glass appearance in lower abdomen?	Meconium ileus; diagnosis and treatment is gastrograffin enema which draws fluid and dissolves pellets
What is the diagnosis of 3 week old baby with non-bilious vomiting?	Congenital hypertrophic pyloric stenosis Diagnose with sonography Treat with surgery (Ramstedt pyloromyotomy) and correct metabolic alkalosis Might be associated with eythromycin
What is the diagnosis of 6-8 week old with increasing conjugated jaundice?	Biliary atresia
How do you diagnose biliary atresia?	HIDA scan after one week of phenobarbital, if no bile in the duodenum do surgery; sweat test and serology is done to rule out other causes
How do you diagnose Hirschprung's disease?	Full thickness biopsy of the rectum
What is the diagnosis of a 9 month old baby with empty	Intussusception

USMLE STEP 3 IN ONE WEEK

RLQ?

When gas gangrene does happen?	Usually 3 days after deep penetrating or dirty wound
How quickly should you operated on open fractures?	
	Within 6h but new data shows up to 24h
What is the one important action in facial injury?	Cervical spine X-ray
What view is needed in posterior shoulder dislocation?	Axillary view
What is the diagnosis if the arm is externally rotated and there is numbness over the deltoid?	Anterior dislocation of the shoulder
What are the differentials for shoulder pain?	Rotator cuff tear or inflammation, biceps tendinitis, osteoarthritis of shoulder joint, frozen shoulder
Where is the rotator cuff pain?	Lateral shoulder area
What is Colles's fracture?	Distal radius fracture with posterior displacement
What is Monteggia fracture?	Fracture of ulna plus radial head dislocation
What is Galeazzi fracture?	Fracture of radius and radiounlar dislocation
What should you do if you are not sure about scaphoid fracture?	Repeat X-ray in 7-10 days

What is the treatment of femoral neck fracture?	Replace the head
What is De Quervain and its best initial treatment?	Tendinitis of exterior pollicis brevis and abductor pollicis longus
What do you do in posterior dislocation of hip?	Emergency reduction
What are the causes of avascular necrosis of hip?	Trauma, steroids, SLE, HIV, SCA, alcohol, decompression sickness, renal diseases, mucopolysacharidosis,
When do you see collateral ligament injury?	Blow to the opposite side of the collateral ligament (Cast if only one injured and surgery if multiple ligaments involved)
What is the significance of anterior and posterior drawer signs?	Cruciate ligaments ruptures; treat arthroscopically in young patients and in old ones use immobilization and rehabilitation
How do you treat meniscal injury?	Arthroscopic menisectomy or repair
What is the next step in the management of stress fracture if it doesn't show on X-ray?	Repeat X-ray in 2 weeks
What is the diagnosis of a patient complaining of popping and limping of the foot with history of quinolones?	Achilles tendon rupture; treat with surgical repair if complete tear plus cast in plantar flexion

What is the least common finding in compartment syndrome?	Pulselessness is uncommon and paralysis is a late sign
How do you diagnose compartment syndrome?	Diagnosis is clinical (passive stretch pain or pain out of proportion) unless mental status not reliable otherwise tissue pressure > 30 or within 20-30 of diastolic pressure)
What do you do if there is pain at the site of the cast?	You must open the cast to rule out compartment syndrome if there is pain on passive movement or toes
How do you treat compartment syndrome?	Emergent fasciotomy
How can compartment syndrome cause acute renal failure?	By causing rhabdomyolysis
When do you do prophylactic fasciotomy?	If there is damage to popliteal artery due to posterior dislocation of knee and reduction is delayed
When do you perform surgery for the back pain?	If there is cauda equina syndrome: bowel/bladder incontinence, flaccid anal sphincter, saddle anesthesia
When isn't MRI helpful for the back pain?	In a typical case of disc herniation in a young patient with severe sudden onset of back pain following moving heavy objects and SLR is positive
Can HLA B27 be used for ankylosing spondylitis?	No
Which tumors have osteoblastic metastasis?	Prostate, breast
Which tumors have lytic metastasis to the bone?	Lung, breast, thyroid and renal

When do you use bone scan in metastasis?	In early diseases it is the most sensitive but MRI is good for neurological signs
What do you see on X-ray of plantar fasciitis?	Spur, no surgery is needed but it takes many months to heal
What are the causes of acute scrotal pain?	Torsion of testis or appendix of testis and epididymitis
What is the one test the must be done if there is clinical diagnosis of orchitis?	Ultrasonography of testis to rule out torsion
How do you treat testicular torsion?	Bilateral orchiopexy
How do you manage acute obstruction of urinary tract + infection kidney?	Emergent decompression by stent, percutaneous nephrostomy otherwise rapid destruction of kidneys and sepsis and finally death can occur
How do you diagnose posterior urethral valve?	Voiding cystourethrogram
What is the diagnosis to be ruled out if the child is having hematuria following trivial trauma?	Urologic congenital anomaly must be ruled out
What is the management of vesicoureteral reflux?	Long term antibiotic prophylaxis until the kid grows out of it
What is the diagnosis if the child is urinating into vagina and they are always wet?	Low implantation of ureter
What is the diagnosis if after hard work there is cold hand	Subclavian steal syndrome: atherosclerosis of the origin of subclavian

with pins and needles?	artery
How do you manage abdominal aortic aneurysm?	>5 cm: if no symptoms do elective surgery, if some symptoms urgent surgery and if severe back pain emergent surgery Between 4-5 cm needs annual ultrasonography
How do you manage arterial embolization of the extremities?	Doppler, thrombolytics if early diagnosis, embolectomy + fasciotomy if late

Pediatrics

What do you need to do for every newborn at delivery?	V.K injection and silver nitrate/ erythromycin ointment
What do you need to do for every newborn before discharge?	Screen for hearing, PKU, hypothyroidism and galactosemia
Does Apgar score predict the outcome?	No
What is the diagnosis of yellow white papules/pustules with erythematous base which peaks on the 2nd day of life?	Erythema toxicum which is self-limited
What is port wine stains?	They are vascular malformations associated with AV malformation, Sturge-Weber disease ; treat them with pulse laser
What is the fate of hemangiomas in newborns?	Mostly they disappear around the age of 5-9. If in the larynx it can cause obstruction, they can cause high output cardiac failure; Treat with steroids or pulse laser
What ear anomalies are associated with?	Renal and genitourinary
What do you see coloboma with?	CHARGE: coloboma, heart, choanal atresia, mental retardation, genitourinary problems and ear anomalies
What syndrome is seen with aniridia?	Wilm's tumor

What trisomies can have omphalocele?	Trisomy 13,18,21
What do you have to check for if three is thyroglossal duct cyst?	Possible to see ectopic thyroid
What is the diagnosis of lateral neck cyst?	Branchial cleft cyst
What do you see with gastroschisis?	Intestinal atresia
What is the main risk associated with undescended testes?	After the first year risk of malignancy is increased
What other anomalies are seen with undescended testes?	Inguinal hernia, hypospadias
When is best to operate on indirect inguinal hernia in a newborn?	Within the first few months of life
What are the main clinical features of infant of diabetic mother?	Macrosomy, low calcium, magnesium, glucose and high birirubin and polycythemia
What anomalies are associated with IODM?	Small left colon and cardiac anomalies including septal hypertrophy (due to hyperinsulinemia and is self-limited), ASD, VSD, Tricuspid atresia)
What is the risk of obesity in children with IODM?	High risk
What is the best initial test for a newborn with respiratory distress syndrome?	CXR: atelectasis, ground glass appearance and air bronchogram; other tests come later (ABG, blood culture,

	CBC, glucose, cranial ultrasonography to rule out intracranial bleeding
How do you manage RDS?	O2, antibiotics, nasal CPAP and surfactant
What is the next step in RDS if hypoxia doesn't improve with O2?	Evaluate cardiac diseases
What is the diagnosis in a premature baby with tachypnea, nasal grunting, and intercostal retraction?	Respiratory distress syndrome (hypoxia, hypercapnia and respiratory acidosis
What is the most accurate test for RDS in a newborn?	L/S ration in amniotic fluid before birth
What are the differentials for RDS?	Pneumonia and if in doubt give antibiotics
What is the most effective treatment for RDS?	Surfactant
What is the primary prevention of RDS?	Antenatal beclomethasone between 34th week to the day before delivery , tocolysis
What are the complications of RDS?	Retinopathy, bronchopulmonary dysplasia, intraventricular hemorrhage
How do you treat transient tachypnea of newborns?	O2
What do you see on X-ray of transient tachypnea of newborns?	Fluid in the fissures, air trapping and perihilar streaking with mild cardiomegaly
What is the diagnosis of a term	Meconium aspiration

infant with severe respiratory distress and possible history of intrauterine fetal distress?

What do you see on X-ray of meconium aspiration?	Over aeration (flat diaphragm, increased AP diameter)and patchy infiltration
How do you treat meconium aspiration?	PPV (positive pressure ventilation) , HFV (high frequency ventilation), ECMO (extracorporal membrane oxygenation), NO (nitrous oxide)
What are the differentials of tachypnea in a newborn?	RDS, meconium aspiration, TTN, pneumonia, diaphragmatic hernia
How do you prevent meconium aspiration prevention?	Intubation and airway suction
What are the complications of meconium aspiration?	Pulmonary hypertension, pneumothorax or pneumomediastinum, aspiration pneumonitis
Where is the obstruction in meconium ileus?	Lower ileum obstruction and usually the cause is cystic fibrosis
What is meconium plug?	Lower colon obstruction and the cause can be cysic fibrosis, Hirschprung's, small left colon as seen in IODM and drug abuse
How do you treat meconium ileus?	Gastrograffin
What is VACTERL?	Vertebra, anal, cardiac, tracheoesophageal fistula, renal, radius and limb anomalies

USMLE STEP 3 IN ONE WEEK

What are the four causes of double bubble syndrome?	Duodenal atresia (Down's syndrome), malrotation, annular pancreas, volvulus
What is Coomb's reagent?	IgM against IgG which is attached to RBC and we detect IgG
What is considered pathologic jaundice?	1st day jaundice, 5 mg bilirubin increase/day, 12 mg bilirubin, 2 mg direct bilirubin, after 2nd week of life
What are the main causes of jaundice in a newborn?	Physiologic (indirect) & pathologic (direct or indirect)
What are the causes of direct pathologic jaundice?	Sepsis, TORCH, TPN, hypothyroidism, tyrosinemia, galactosemia, cystic fibrosis, choledochal cyst
What are the causes of indirect pathologic jaundice?	Breast mild jaundice (2nd week), breastfeeding failure jaundice (1st week) **Coomb's positive**: Rh, ABO incompatibilities, thalassemia minor **Coomb's negative** and increase Hb: IODM, polycythemia, maternofetal transfusion, delayed cord clamping, IUGR **Coomb's negative and Hb is decreased or normal**: hereditary spherocytosis or elliptocytosis, G6PD or pyruvate kinase deficiency
What is the workup for neonatal jaundice?	CBC, bilirubin, ret. , LDH, haptoglobin, direct Coombs, mother and infant blood grouping, urinalysis and culture
What is jaundice happens after at least 2 weeks of life?	If direct jaundice: cholestatic jaundice therefore LFT, ultrasonography and biopsy

	If indirect jaundice: conjugation disorders (Gilbert, CNS I and II), hemolysis, enzyme or membrane defects in RBC, UTI and other infections
How do you manage kernicterus?	Immediate exchange transfusion and if bilirubin> 12 use phototherapy
Do you need to do LP in any case of sepsis?	LP isn't part of sepsis evaluation unless meningitis is suspected
What are the causes of neonatal sepsis?	1st 24h: pneumonia by E coli, GBS, Listeria, HiB If later: meningitis, sepsis by Staph., E coli, Klebsiella and Pseudomona
How do you treat neonatal sepsis?	If no meningitis suspected ampicillin + gentamicin until 72h culture is negative; if meningitis suspected use ampicillin and cefotaxime
What kind of problem can be seen with ceftriaxone in newborns?	Rare cases of calcium ppt. with ceftriaxone, also displaces bilirubin from albumin (kern icterus)
What are the causes of TORCH syndrome?	1. Toxoplasmosis: IgM, calcified Chorioretinitis 2. Rubella: IgM, cardiac, cataract, deafness 3. CMV: urine culture, periventricular calcification, microcephaly, petechial & low platelets 4. Herpes: Tzanck and PCR; 1st week (pneumonia & shock), 2nd week (vesicles and keratoconjunctivitis); 3rd week (meningoencephalitis) 5. Others: varicella (IgM and PCR of amniotic fluid) syphilis(

	VDRL)
How do you workup neonatal seizure?	1. Physical exam: ocular deviation doesn't go away with stimulus 2. EEG (maybe normal) 3. CBC, glucose, Ca, Mg, Na, P; amino acid assay and urinary organic acids 4. Cord blood IgM 5. Blood and urine culture 6. If preterm ultrasonography of head (IVH)
What is the diagnosis of a newborn with fever, diarrhea, vomiting, tachycardia, tachypnea, irritability, hyperactive, seizure, tremor, jitters, nasal stuffiness?	Withdrawal syndrome: it is in the first 48h think of cocaine, heroin, amphetamine, alcohol If it happens from 4-14 days it can be methadone
What are the complications of drug addiction in infants?	Sudden infant death syndrome, IUGR, anomalies, low birth weight
What are the complications of drug addiction in the mother?	Abruption and IVH, breach, STD
How do you treat withdrawal syndrome?	Opioids, phenobarbital, never give naloxone if opioids use suspected in the mother, it can precipitate withdrawal
What is the anomaly caused by valproate or carbamazepine?	Neural tube defects and mental retardation
What is the effect of phenobarbital on vitamin K?	Decrease V.K
What cardiac anomaly is caused by lithium?	Ebstein's: atrialization of right ventricle

What adverse effect is shared between lithium and demeclocycline?	Diabetes insipidus Demeclocycline can be used to treat SIADH but lithium is not used due to its toxicity
What medication can cause facial anomalies?	ACE inhibitors, phenytoin, isotretinoin, warfarin
What are the main features of Down's syndrome?	Speckling of iris, endocardial cushion defect, tracheoesophageal fistula, duodenal atresia, hypothyroidism, ALL, Alzheimer's
What are the main features of trisomy 18?	Heart &renal anomalies and index finger is over the 3rd finger ; they die mostly in the 1st year
What are the main features of trisomy 13?	Patau syndrome: midface &forebrain anomaly, cleft lip/palate, head, renal, single artery
What is WAGR?	Wilm's, aniridia, genitourinary and mental retardation
What are the main features of Kleinfelter's?	XXY, low IQ, gynecomastia, low testosterone level, hypogoandism, hypovirilism; treatment is testosterone replacement
What are the main features of Turner's?	XO genotype, low IQ, horseshoe kidney, aortic coarctation, bicuspid valve, hypothyroidism; treatment is estrogen, growth hormone and anabolic steroids
What is fragile X syndrome?	The most common cause of mental retardation in boys, large ears, large testes, small head
What is Beckwith-	IGF-2 is disrupted, multiorgan

Weidemann?	enlargement (macrosomia, macroglossia, hyperplasia of beta cells causing hypoglycemia, increased RBC number causing polycythemia, large kidneys, increase risk of abdominal tumors (Wilm's, hapatoblastoma)
What is Prader Willi syndrome?	Obesity, small genitalia, mental retardation, binge eating; deletion of paternal part of chromosome
What is Angleman syndrome?	Deletion of maternal part of chromosome as seen in Prader- Willi; happy puppet syndrome, epilepsy
What are the main features of fetal alcohol syndrome?	Mandibular hypoplasia, cleft palate, monitor airway because of obstruction in the first 4 weeks of life
What is the significant of height at 2 years of age?	Best predictor of height
What are the normal heights at 6 months or one year of age?	At 6 months should be doubled and at one year tripled
What is the best indicator of acute malnutrition?	Weight divided by height is <5th percentile
What is the best indicator for normal weight?	BMI
What is the relationship between skeletal and sexual maturity?	They should match
What is the most common cause of failure to thrive?	Psychological deprivation

What is the first thing that you should do when you see an underfed child?	Child protective services should be informed
What is the next step if a child crosses two major growth percentiles?	Workup is necessary
What is the hallmark of short stature because of constitutional delay?	Growth velocity is normal and is parallel to the graphs
What are the differentials if both weight and height is low?	Systemic diseases: CRP,EST,CBC,LFT,BUN,Cr. Genetic short stature: normal bone age Constitutional delay: delayed bone age
What are the differentials if weight is normal and height is low?	Low growth hormone, low T4, high cortisol, skeletal dysplasia
What are the differentials if weight is severely low and height is mildly low?	Malabsorption, malnutrition; tests which are helpful are fecal fat and sweat chloride test
What are the breast-feeding contraindications?	HIV, CMV, HSV (if breast lesion), HBV (until vaccinated), substance abuse, TB & sepsis (unless the baby has it), drugs (Li, iodide, smoking, chemotherapy), breast cancer
What are the drugs which are relatively contraindicated in breast feeding?	Metronidazole, tetracycline, sulfa, sedatives, neuroleptics and steroids
What reflexes are going to disappear after 4-6 months?	Tonic neck, Moro's, grasp, rooting and placing

USMLE STEP 3 IN ONE WEEK

When does parachute reflex appears?	6-8 months and stays forever
At what age can the infant do 3, 4 and 7 cube towers?	15, 18 and 24 months of age.
What is considered enuresis?	At least twice a week for at least 3 months in child> 5 years old
What is the workup for enuresis?	Urinalysis initially, culture if signs of infection, if recurrent infection do ultrasonography or VCUG
How do you treat enuresis?	Best initial treatment is alarm therapy; never punish the child; behavioral therapy and if it fails use desmopressin and finally TCA
What is encopresis?	Involuntary or intentional defecation in inappropriate setting; it can be retentive (constipation and overflow incontinence) or non-retentive (seen in abuse also)
Is a reaction to DPT including fever, redness and sore throat considered as contraindication to DPT?	No
Is family history of seizure or sudden infant death syndrome a contraindication to vaccination?	NO
Can you give MMR to someone with egg allergy?	Yes
What vaccines can you not	

give to someone with egg allergy?	Flu and yellow fever
Is there any relation between MMR and autism or IBD?	None
Is there any relation between hepatitis B vaccine and demyelinating diseases?	None
What vaccine is given at birth, one month and 6 months?	Hepatitis B
What vaccines are given at 2, 4, 6 months?	DTaP, HiB, Rota, IPV, PCV
When do give MMR?	15 months and 4-6 years
What vaccines are given at 4-6 years?	DTaP, IPV, MMR
What vaccines are given at 11-12 years?	HPV (3 doses), TdaP, MCV4 (meningococcal)
What is the management after exposure to measles?	Only immunoglobulins: under 6 months, pregnant or immunocompromised Ig + vaccination: 6-12 months of age Vaccine: > 1 year old and only if within 3 days of exposure
How do you manage exposure to varicella?	VZIG plus vaccine (except for pregnant and newborns who get only VZIG) Note: newborns must have mothers who got varicella 5 days before to 2 days after delivery
What do you do for exposure	None

to mumps or rubella?	
What do you do if mother is HBsAg positive?	Ig within 12h of delivery plus first dose of vaccine given at 2 different sites of injection
After the first five doses of DTaP when do you give pertussis booster?	During adolescence
When do you give Td (tetanus booster)?	At 11 and every 10 years after that
Do you give HiB vaccine after 5 years?	Not given
Can varicella vaccine prevent shingles?	Herpes zoster is seen even after immunization
When do you give meningococcal vaccine?	At 11, all college freshmen in dorms
What kind of workup do you do for child abuse?	Coagulation studies, if severe injury perform CT of head and possibly MRI, eye exam, if abdominal trauma: LFT, amylase, lipase, stool and urine for blood, CT abdomen
When do you hospitalize a case of child abuse?	Medical reasons, no safe place, diagnosis not clear
How do you manage a case of child abuse?	First manage medical and surgical issues then report to CPS (child protective services) by phone and in 48h report
What are the main features of croup?	Barking cough, stridor, parainfluenza and influenza are the causes
What are the main features of	Epiglottitis: toxic appearance, sitting in

epiglottitis?	tripod position, dysphagia, stridor
What are the main features of tracheitis?	No dysphagia, brassy cough, no drooling, subglottis narrowed, no stridor,
What do you have to rule out in a child under 3 and recurrent infection?	Foreign body
What is the most common cause of bronchiolitis?	RAP: RSV, Adenovirus, Parainfluenza
18 months old boy with fever, wheezing, cough, apnea, dyspnea, CXR shows hyperinflation and patchy atelectasis, what is the diagnosis?	Bronchiolitis
How do you diagnose bronchiolitis?	Best initial test is CXR, however immunofluorescence of nasopharyngeal swab is the most specific
What is the treatment of bronchiolitis?	Supportive
How do you prevent bronchiolitis?	RSV IVIG or palivizumab for high risk patients
What are the most common cause of pneumonia in a child less than 5 and more than 5 years of age?	<5 is viral mostly RSV; >5 is bacterial (Strep. pneumonia, mycoplasma, chlamydia)
In what age group Chlamydia trachomatis can cause pneumonia?	1-3 months

What is the diagnosis of a 6 weeks old baby with staccato cough, eosinophilia, conjunctivitis and hyperinflation of the lungs?	Chlamydia trachomatis, treat with 14 days of erythromycin
How high is the level of WBC in bacterial pneumonia?	15,000 to 40,000
What is the usual level of WBC in viral pneumonia?	< 20,000
How do you diagnose mycoplasma infection?	IgM titer and blood culture (just to rule out other causes)
Is there any indication for sputum culture in children suspected of pneumonia?	None
How do you treat pneumonia in children?	Outpatient: amoxicillin and clavulanate; inpatient: cefuroxime (add vancomycin if Staph. is suspected)
What is the usual level of WBC in viral pneumonia?	< 20,000
How do you diagnose mycoplasma infection?	IgM titer and blood culture (just to rule out other causes)
Is there any indication for sputum culture in children suspected of pneumonia?	None
How do you treat pneumonia in children?	Outpatient: amoxicillin and clavulanate; inpatient: cefuroxime (add vancomycin if Staph. is suspected)
What is cefuroxime?	A 2nd generation cephalosporin which is effective for sinopulmonary infections

What percentage of viral infections has bacterial infection at the same time in children?	30%
What level of sweat chloride test is significant?	If >60 mEq/lit then cystic fibrosis is suspected so repeat the test once more
What is the most common presentation of cystic fibrosis?	Meconium ileus; also other presentations like: malabsorption and failure to thrive, infertility, chronic cough and mucus, rectal prolapse, allergic bronchopulmonary aspergillosis
What genetic testing do you do for cystic fibrosis?	Chromosome 7 is tested for a defect but not all cases are detected; it is good for prenatal diagnosis
How do you screen for cystic fibrosis?	Immunoreactive trypsinogen in blood; however sweat test and DNA probes are the most accurate ones
How do you treat cystic fibrosis pneumonia?	Vanco + tobramycin + piperacillin-tazobactam
What is the treatment for cystic fibrosis?	Supportive: albuterol or saline aerosol, chest physiotherapy, ibuprofen might help lungs, pancrelipase Treat the infection
When do you call a murmur an innocent murmur?	If it is a II/VI systolic murmur
Are expectorant like guaifenesin effective in cystic fibrosis?	No
What are the acyanotic congenital heart diseases?	VSD, ASD, AV canal, pulmonary stenosis, PDA, aortic stenosis, aortic coarctation
What are the cyanotic	TTTT: tetralogy of Fallot, transposition

USMLE STEP 3 IN ONE WEEK

congenital heart diseases?	of great arteries, tricuspid atresia, total anomalous pulmonary veins return
What are the four defects seen in tetralogy of Fallot?	PROV: pulmonary stenosis, RVH, Overriding of aorta, VSD
How reassuring is the antenatal ultrasound for diagnosing heart defects?	Not at all
Right to left shunt usually manifest around which months of age?	2-6 months after birth
Why do you give antibiotics when you suspect congenital heart diseases?	It looks like sepsis
When does a PDA dependent congenital heart disease show?	Within the first one month of life
What is the best initial test for CHD?	CXR, EKG
What is the most specific test for CHD?	Ultrasonography
What percentage of VSD closes in the first 6 months?	Half of them
What is the significance of a loud murmur in VSD?	VSD is small
When do you operate on VSD?	When failure to thrive, pulmonary hypertension, right to left shunt >2:1
How many different types of ASD do we have?	Septum primum, septum secundum and endocardial cushion defect
Which type of ASD is the most	Septum secundum; it closes by the end

common one?	of 4th year
Which type of ASD needs surgery?	Primum and sinus venousus
What is patent foramen ovale?	Short flap defect caused by excessive resorption of septum primum
What is high septal defect?	Sinus venousus type
What is the diagnosis of loud S1, wide fixed splitting of S2, systolic ejection murmur on left sternal border?	ASD
Why do we see ejection murmur in ASD?	Overflow through pulmonary valve
How do you treat pulmonary stenosis?	PGE1 and angioplasty
What is the most common form of aortic coarctation?	Post ductal stenosis, 98% is at the origin of subclavian artery
How do you treat tetralogy of Fallot?	O2, beta blockers, PGE1 if cyanotic at birth, surgery after 4-12 months
When do you give antibiotic prophylaxis for congenital heart diseases?	History of endocarditis, mechanical valves, CHD if unrepaired or repaired with persistent defect, cardiac transplantation with valve defect
What percentile is considered hypertension in children?	>95 percentile
When and how do you check blood pressure in children for the first time?	At 3 years old four limbs

USMLE STEP 3 IN ONE WEEK

When do you need to do a workup for hypertension in children? — Always

What are the differentials for hypertension in children?

If at birth think of renal artery stenosis; if early childhood think of renal, coarctation, medications; if during adolescence it could be essential HTN, renovascular, glomerulonephritis, HSP, HUS, ATN, leukemia

How do you treat severe hypertension in children? — ACE inhibitors plus calcium channel blockers if severe otherwise diuretics or beta blockers

What is the diagnosis if after 5-10 days of infection a child has anemia, oliguria, acute renal failure and low platelets? — HUS (hemolytic uremic syndrome)

What is the most common cause of renal failure in children?

HUS

How do you treat hemolytic uremic syndrome? — Treat HTN, early dialysis, aggressive nutritional treatment

What presentation is seen if malrotation is causing incomplete obstruction? — Giardia

What is the best initial therapy for GERD in children? — Change of feeding technique and thickening of food

What are the 2nd and 3rd lines — H2 blockers and proton pump

of therapy for GERD in children?	inhibitors; if very severe fundoplication
What is the cause of acute small bowel obstruction and no history of bowel surgery?	Volvulus must be ruled out
What is the best initial test for malrotation and volvulus?	Ultrasonography or barium enema
What is the next test in a 2 year old with rectal bleeding?	Tc-99m pertechnetate scan (Meckel scan)
What are the differentials of Meckel's diverticulum?	Appendicitis, diverticulitis, intussusception
What are the causes of intussusception?	Meckel's, HSP, polyp, neurofibroma, hemangiomas
What is the best initial test for intussusception?	Abdominal X-ray to rule out obstruction
What is the best test intussusception for?	Air enema is both diagnostic and therapeutic
Can you give ceftriaxone in neonates with kernicterus?	No
What is the most common age group for UTI in children?	<1 year in male and >2 years in female; peak is during infancy and toilet training
How do you treat UTI in children?	1. Cystitis: ampicillin or Bactrim 2. Pyelonephritis: ampicillin + gentamicin or ceftriaxone + gentamicin

After what age can you give quinolones to children?	After 16
What age group cannot receive sulfonamide or nitrofurantoin?	Less than 1 year old
After what age can you give tetracycline?	After 7
How do you diagnose vesicoureteral reflux?	VCUG and renal scan
	Breakthrough UTI, new scars, failure to resolve
How do you follow up UTI in children?	1. Urine culture one week after stopping antibiotics 2. Follow up for 1-2 years 3. VCUG & ultrasonography in all males / females less than 5 of > 5 and recurrent infection/ UTI + fever
What is the most common cause of bladder obstruction in male children?	Posterior urethral valve
What is the most common cause of abdominal mass in children?	Hydronephrosis and polycyctic kidney disease
What is the diagnosis in a 5-12 years old 1-2 weeks after pharyngitis or 3-6 weeks after impetigo with high blood pressure, edema and hematuria?	Post streptococcal glomerulonephritis

How do you diagnose PSGN?	Rising titer of ASO + positive culture, anti DNase (the most specific test), low C3, urinalysis
How do you treat PSGN?	Supportive: salt restriction, diuresis, fluid and electrolyte balance, penicillin Note: no need for steroids or antihypertensives
What is the diagnosis of a 25 years old post upper respiratory infection who has gross hematuria, high blood pressure and mild proteinuria with normal C3?	Berger's disease (IgA nephropathy) which is the most common cause of chronic glomerulonephritis
A boy with sensorineural hearing loss, isolated hematuria and ocular symptoms has what diagnosis?	Alport's syndrome
What is the mode of inheritance in infantile PCKD?	Autosomal recessive
How do you treat infantile PCKD?	Dialysis and transplantation
What are the causes of transient proteinuria?	CDEF: cold, dehydration, exercise, fever
What level of proteinuria is glomerular?	>1 g /day
What is the most common	Focal segmental glumerulosclerosis (

cause of nephrotic syndrome? What is the diagnosis of nephrotic syndrome in a 2-6 year old following an infection?	50% of cases in African Americans) MCD (minimal chain disease); treat typical cases with steroids and no biopsy needed
How do you treat relapsing MCD?	Cyclophosphamide, cyclosporine, high dose of pulse prednisone
What are the main compilations of nephrotic syndrome?	Subacute bacterial peritonitis, thromboembolism
What is the best test for 21 hydroxylase deficiency?	17 hydroxyprogesterone before and after ACTH test
How do you treat CAH due to 21 hydroxylase deficiency?	Hydrocortisone, fludrocortisone, surgery
What is the level of platelets in Kawasaki disease?	It can be > 100,000, also CRP and ESR are high
How do you treat Kawasaki disease?	High dose aspirin + IVIG and anticoagulation if platelets are very high
When do coronary diseases happen in Kawasaki disease?	During 2nd or 3rd week
What is the typical age for Kawasaki disease?	Mostly <5
When do you do Echo in Kawasaki disease?	Baseline, during 2nd or 3rd week, finally during 6-8 weeks
What is the typical age for HSP?	2-8 years old
What is the pathogenesis of	IgA + complement deposits and causes

HSP?	vasculitis in skin, kidney, GI, joint and can cause intussusception
What is the diagnosis of a 4 year old with high platelets, anemia, high ESR (IgM and IgA are high); anticardiolipin and antiphospholipid Ab are increased?	HSP (Henoch- Schonline Purpura)
How do you treat HSP?	Aspirin if anti phospholipid Ab present, steroids if renal/GI involvement, supportive treatment for all
When is Hb nadir in full term infants?	12th week
When is Hb nadir in perterms?	3-6 week
For how long are iron stores enough in newborns?	4-6 months
What is the most common age for iron deficiency anemia in pediatrics?	9-24 months of age
For how long do you treat iron deficiency anemia?	8 weeks after normal lab values
What is the diagnosis of a child with ADHD, constipation, mental changes and impaired growth?	Lead poisoning
What is the normal BLL (blood lead level)?	<10 is normal; >15 has to be reported; > 45 needs chelating agents
What are the main lab findings in lead poisoning?	MCV & MCHC are low, basophilic stippling, free erythrocyte porphyrin is

	high, X-ray of bones show dense lead lines
What is the most common cause of death in sickle anemia?	Infection, acute chest syndrome, acute splenic sequestration (peak is 6 months to 3 years)
How do you manage actue chest syndrome?	IV fluid, azithromycin and ceftriaxone, morphine
When do you transfuse blood in sickle cell anemia?	Before surgery; symptomatic anemia (shortness of breath, chest pain); life threatening complication (stroke, splenic sequestration, acute chest syndrome)
Do you transfuse a sickle cell anemia patient who has recurrent painful attacks?	No
What are the indications of hydroxyurea?	More than 3 crisis per year, symptomatic anemia, life threatening complications
When do you give penicillin prophylaxis in sickle cell anemia?	At 2 months of age up to 5 years of age
What kind of vaccination is recommended for sickle cell anemia?	Pneumococcus (at 2 months), meningitis (at 2 years), influenza every 6 months
What is the only definite treatment of sickle cell anemia?	Bone marrow transplantation
What are the best initial and the most specific test for thalassemia major?	Hb electrophoresis
When do you perform	At 5 years of age

splenectomy in thalassemia major?	
How do you treat thalassemia major?	Transfusion, deferoxamine, splenectomy and vaccination, folate replacement, growth hormone, bone marrow transplantation
How do you manage a 9 year old boy with well controlled hemophilia who suddenly develops bleeding?	Mixing studies shows uncorrected which means anticoagulation factor Ab has developed. If partially corrected it means there is some inhibitor like heparin. If it is corrected then it is factor deficiency
What is the diagnosis if PTT is high; mixing studies is abnormal but no clinical bleeding?	Lupus anticoagulant
What is Bernard Soulier's disease?	GP Ib (a receptor for vWF) is deficient
What is Glanzmann's thromboasthenia?	GP IIb/IIIa (receptor for ADP) is deficient
How do you treat hemophilia?	If mild: desmopressin + either aminocaproic acid or tranexamic acid If major bleeding: F VIII replacement
Why do we need smear in a typical case of ITP?	To rule out HUS or TTP
How do you treat ITP?	1st Prednisone, then IVIG and finally splenectomy if chronic
What is the relationship between febrile seizure and epilepsy?	No relationship unless it is >15 minutes, > one per day, focal neurologic findings, before 9 months old and positive family

	history, abnormal development, pre-existing neurologic disease
How do you diagnose epilepsy?	At least 2 attacks 24h apart or one attack plus positive EEG
When do you stop medication in epilepsy?	If no seizures for 2 years
How do you diagnose and treat absence seizure?	Diagnosis: history and 3 second spikes + generalized wave discharge Treatment: ethosuximide or valproate
What is juvenile myoclonic epilepsy and how do you treat it?	Jerky movement in the morning; spikes and slow waves on EEG, treat with valproate
What is the earliest sign of phenytoin toxicity?	Lateral nystagmus
What are the main features of infantile spasm?	Clusters of mixed spasms of the trunk and extremities for minutes ; 70 % have nervous system diseases, associated with Down syndrome, very high voltage slow waves and spikes on EEG; Treat with ACTH, prednisone, vigabatrin, B6, valproate or carbamazepine
How do you treat partial seizures?	Valproate
How do you treat generalized seizures?	All seizures except for absence and infantile spasm
When can you use valproate in children?	Lasts < 1 week in children < 3 years, at least 38 degrees
What is the definition of fever	In neonates: admit, culture and

without a focus in pediatrics?	antibiotics for GEL (Group B Strep, E coli and Listeria)
How do you manage fever without a focus?	In infants: if toxic IV antibiotics; if well appearing single dose of IM ceftriaxone
Can you use IV dexamethasone for HiB meningitis?	There is proven effect
How do you treat meningitis empirically?	Vancomycin + ceftriaxone
How do you treat N. meningitides meningitis in children?	Penicillin for a week
How do you treat Strep pneumonia meningitis in children?	Penicillin and ceftriaxone for 2 weeks
How do you treat HiB meningitis?	Ampicillin plus dexamethasone
How do you treat G- meningitis in children?	3 weeks of any 3rd generation cephalosporins
What is the most common complication of meningitis?	Hearing loss
What is the diagnosis of persistent fever + seizure after meningitis?	HiB subdural effusion
What are the complications if you treat meningitis late?	Mental retardation, thrombosis, neurologic dysfunction
What are the Neisseria	DIC, adrenal hemorrhage , heart and

complications?	renal failure
What infection gets prophylactic rifampin?	Only for Neisseria and HiB infection

Obstetrics & Gynecology

What do we mean by parity?	Birth after 24 weeks of gestation
What are the suggestive signs of pregnancy?	Amenorrhea, large uterus, high beta hCG
What do confirm pregnancy?	1. Presence of gestational sac with transvaginal ultrasonography around 4-5 weeks) 2. Fetal heart motion 5-6 week by ultrasound or fetal heart sounds around 8-10 week by Doppler 3. Fetal movement around 20th week by the examiner
What are the pregnancy screening tests?	CBC, U/A, ABO, Rh, Coombs (direct and indirect), VDRL, rubella and toxoplasma titers, HBsAg, HIV, Pap smear
What is considered anemia in pregnancy?	Hb<10
What is considered leukocytosis in pregnancy?	WBC>16000
What is the next step in pregnancy if platelets are <150,000?	Rule out HELLP (hemolysis, elevated liver enzymes, low platelets) & ITP (immune thrombocytopenic purpura)

What is the next step if HBsAg is positive in pregnancy?	HBeAg is measured
If an infant is born to HIV positive mother what is the result of ELISA test?	Always positive for ELISA
What are the early screening tests for trisomy 21?	1. Beta hCG 2. Protein A 3. Nuchal translucency Note: confirm with chorionic villous sampling in 1st trimester
What is the most common cause of increased alpha fetoprotein?	Mistake in pregnancy date therefore confirm it with ultrasound
What is triple test plus inhibin?	Beta hCG, alpha fetoprotein, estriol + inhibin, alpha fetoprotein is positive in neural tube defect; inhibin and hCG is high in Down syndrome (E3 & alpha fetoprotein are low)
When do you need to start folate for pregnant women?	One month before pregnancy
What is the next step if maternal serum AFP is decreased?	Amniocentesis for karyotyping
What is the next step if maternal serum AFP is increased?	Amniocentesis for AFP and acetyl choline esterase; if they are both high, NTD is very likely
How do you screen for gestational diabetes?	At 24-28 weeks give 50 gram of glucose for 1h OGTT (oral glucose tolerance test) is positive do 3h 100 g OGTT
How do you screen for group B Strep in pregnancy?	Culture at 35-37 weeks and if positive give intrapartum IV penicillin (if allergic clindamycin)

What is indirect Coombs test?	In Rh negative mothers looks for anti-D Ab (if present don't give Rhogam)
What are the oral GTT values?	1h >140, 2h>155, 3h>180 if any of them abnormal it is impaired glucose tolerance test, if two abnormal it is gestational diabetes
How do you treat nausea and vomiting of pregnancy?	B6, doxylamine (a short acting sedating antihistamine), ondansetrone, promethazine, metoclopramide
What are the indications of Rhogam?	Rh negative mothers at 28 weeks, within 72h of delivery, after abortion, amniocentesis, CVS & heavy vaginal bleeding
What are the causes of painless late vaginal bleeding in pregnancy?	Placenta previa, vasa previa
What is the cause of painful late vaginal bleeding in pregnancy?	Placenta abruption
What do you see on NST if there is loss of blood from fetal circulation?	Late deceleration and bradycardia
How do you manage late pregnancy bleeding?	IV fluid, check vitals frequently, external fetal monitoring, CBC, type and cross match, DIC workup (PT, PTT, D-dimer, fibrinogen), perform ultrasound if no placenta previa perform vaginal exam to rule out laceration; if >36 weeks and fetus is in danger deliver, manage hypovolemia and shock if present

USMLE STEP 3 IN ONE WEEK

What are the causes of placenta abruption?	HTN, Cocaine and trauma
What are placenta accreta, increta, percreta?	Insertion in entire endometrium, myometrium, serosa respectively. Treat with C-section
Can you perform amniotomy if vessels are seen over internal os?	No
What is the triad of vasa previa?	Rupture of membrane, painless bleeding, bradycardia or late deceleration; treat with C-section
What is the diagnosis of sudden onset of pain, loss of fetal heart rate, history of uterine scar?	Uterine rupture
How do you manage abruption or placenta previa?	At 36 weeks or higher perform vaginal delivery as long as placenta is >2 cm away from os Before 34 weeks admit and observe if bleeding stops All other cases need C-section
What do you do if previous birth was complicated by group B Strep sepsis?	Intrapatum IV penicillin G or clindamycin if allergy to penicillin
What percentage of women have group B Strep and are asymptomatic?	30%
When does group B Strep sepsis or pneumonia happen?	Hours or days after birth while meningitis happens after a week
When is antibiotics indicated	Previous infection, positive culture,

in group B Strep?	rupture of membrane >18 weeks, maternal fever, preterm
What if culture was positive for group B Strep in the last pregnancy and now it is negative?	No antibiotic is needed
How do you treat toxoplasmosis?	Pyrimethamine + sulfadiazine
What are the main features of toxoplasmosis?	Chorioretinitis, hydrocephalus, intracranial calcification
How do you prevent transmission of toxoplasmosis?	Spiramycin
What is the management of varicella in pregnancy?	Check Ab level and if it is high enough no treatment is needed
When is the greatest risk for varicella to affect the newborn?	From 5 days before up to 2 days after delivery
When is VZIG indicated?	Within four days of infection
What are the main features of neonatal varicella infection? How do you treat varicella neonatal infection?	Chorioretinitis, cataract, microcephalia, microophthalmia, limb hypoplasia, zigzag skin lesions VZIG + acyclovir
What are the main features of rubella infection?	Cataract, cardiac defects, hearing loss, mental retardation, thrombocytopenia, blueberry muffin rash, hepatosplenomegaly
What is the most common congenital viral infection?	CMV

What are the main clinical features of congenital CMV?	Calcification, microcephaly, cataract very early jaundice, hepatosplenomegaly, IUGR, prematurity & pneumonia
How do you diagnose CMV infection?	Urine culture and if needed PCR
What is the effect of ganciclovir in CMV infection?	Prevents shedding and hearing loss but doesn't cure it
What is the rate of transplacental infection with HSV?	With primary HSV infection during pregnancy 50% chance of transplacental infection, from which 50% die and the rest have: MR, meningoencephalitis, pneumonia, jaundice & hepatosplenomegaly
How do you diagnose HSV infection?	Vesicle fluid culture, PCR of maternal blood (not done routinely)
How do you prevent HSV congenital infection?	C-section, no scalp electrode allowed, manage premature rupture of membrane, avoid kissing neonates, avoid sex if partner has it
What is the next step if there is history of HSV infection during pregnancy?	Start treating at 36 weeks and if there is active infection at term C-section; if there is only history of exposure check IgG and if positive do the same
What are the most effective methods of preventing HIV vertical transmission?	Zidovudine therapy; other methods are: triple therapy, C-section, avoid breastfeeding, and avoid artificial rupture of membrane

USMLE STEP 3 IN ONE WEEK

When do you start with triple therapy in pregnancy?	Start at 14 weeks + intrapartum IV zidovudine Newborn needs zidovudine & Bactrim for 6 weeks
When do you do C-section in HIV positive mothers?	At 38 weeks unless viral load is <1000
Is there any immunity against syphilis infection?	None
What are the features of 1st trimester syphilis?	Huge placenta, hydrops fetalis, anemia, low platelets, hepatosplenomegaly, maculopapular rash
What is the chance of transplacental infection in primary or secondary syphilis?	60%
What are the main features of late pregnancy syphilis?	MDHSS: mulberry molars, deafness, Hutchinson's teeth, saddle nose, saber shin
How do you diagnose syphilis?	VDRL, FTA-ABS, MHA-TP (microhemagglutination)
What percentage of neonates with HBV does develop chronic liver disease?	80%
What are the contraindications to breast feeding?	HHHH-TB & Drugs: HIV, HBV, HSV on breast, HTLV-1, TB, alcohol, smoking, cytotoxic drugs, child conditions don't allow it e.g. galactosemia
What is HELLP syndrome?	Hemolysis, elevated liver enzymes, low

	platelets
Who should receive HBV vaccine?	All HBsAg negative pregnants should have it.
Who should receive HBIG?	Post exposure prophylaxis
What is the management of neonates with hepatitis B infection?	Both vaccine and HBIG should be given
What is the difference between chronic HTN versus gestational hypertension?	If before 20 weeks it is chronic and if after that is gestational
What is severe pre-eclampsia?	Proteinuria and warning signs: headache, epigastric pain, blurred vision, pulmonary embolism, oliguria, HELLP
What is mild eclampsia?	HTN, proteinuria and edema
What are the risk factors for pre-eclampsia?	Extreme age, multiple pregnancy, GTD (mole), chronic HTN, diabetes, chronic renal disease, primipara
What is the mechanism of seizure in eclampsia?	Vasospasm in the brain causing seizure
Are seizure disorders a risk factor for developing pre-eclampsia?	No
What are the lab findings in pre-eclampsia?	Proteinuria, DIC & HELLP, hemoconcentration (increased Hct,BUN,Cr. & UA)

How do you treat pre-eclampsia or eclampsia?	Control BP with hydralazine, seizure with MgSO4, deliver and monitor
How do you control BP in pre-eclampsia?	goal is 140-150/90-100 ; use methyldopa or second line is beta blockers but risk of IUGR; if severe use hydralazine or labetolol
How do you control seizure in eclampsia?	MgSO4 IV bolus for treatment and infusion for prophylaxis
How do you monitor pre-eclampsia?	Serial monitoring with ultrasound, BP measurement and urine protein
How do you manage labor & delivery in pre-eclampsia?	At 36 weeks with mild proteinuria induce the labor, if case is severe prompt delivery
Can HELLP happen postpartum?	Within 2 days of postpartum can happen
What are the risk factors for HELLP?	Old, multigravida, white
How do you manage HELLP?	Delivery at any gestational age, MgSO4, dexamethasone if platelets < 100,000 or if premature, platelets if <20,000 or 50,000 if C-section needed
What are the complications of HELLP?	DIC, abruption, fetal demise, hepatic rupture
Is there any use for steroids in HELLP?	< 36 for lung maturation, >36 for low platelets
What percentage of maternal death is due to cardiac diseases?	10% of all deaths in pregnancy
When is the maximum stress	28-34 weeks

on the heart during pregnancy?

Which cardiac diseases are contraindications to pregnancy?	Pulmonary hypertension, Eisenmenger syn., severe valve diseases, postpartum cardiomyopathy
When does peripartum cardiomyopathy happen?	One month before to 5 months after delivery; more in multiple gestation, multipara, pre-eclampsia No other causes of CMP is present
How do you manage heart failure during pregnancy?	beta blockers, nitrates and furosemide
What is the management if there is rheumatic heart disease in a pregnant woman?	Daily antibiotic prophylaxis
Does uncomplicated vaginal delivery in valvular heart diseases need antibiotics?	No antibiotic prophylaxis needed
Which one of stenotic or regurgitant valvular diseases are worse in pregnancy?	Stenotic is worse
What are the hypercoagulable states in pregnancy which need anticoagulation?	Pulmonary embolism (leading cause of maternal death in the US) DVT, A. fib + underlying heart disease, antiphospholipid syndrome, severe heart failure, Eisenmenger syndrome
How do you give anticoagulation in pregnancy?	LMWH throughout pregnancy; heparin during labor and delivery, warfarin for 6 weeks after delivery
What are the advantages of LMWH?	Will not cross placenta and won't cause osteopenia

USMLE STEP 3 IN ONE WEEK

What is the difference between miscarriage and stillbirth?

>24 weeks is still birth, <20-24 weeks is abortion

How do you treat hyperthyroidism in pregnancy?

Beta blockers

How do you treat hypothyroidism in pregnancy?

Hormone replacement

What is the use of PTU in pregnancy?

It is the 1st line in pregnancy for Graves' disease but it can pass placenta and cause goiter & hypothyroidism in newborns

What are the blood sugar values in non- pregnant women?

<100 is normal, 100-125 is pre-diabetic, >125 is diabetes

What are the blood sugar values in pregnant women?

Target is <90 fasting blood glucose, <120 1h after a meal is also the target

How do you manage gestational diabetes?

Only diet

How do you manage diabetes in pregnancy?

Insulin

What is the danger of hypoglycemia in breast feeding mothers?

Hypoglycemia in neonate

How do you treat Trichomonas in breast feeding mother?
How do you monitor diabetes in pregnancy?

Single dose of 2 g metronidazole and resume breast feeding the next day
HbA1c is tested and if it is high do fetal echo around 22-24 weeks or ultrasound around 18-20 weeks   check triple markers around 16-18 weeks monthly ultrasound with biophysical

	profile weekly NST & AFI at 32 weeks unless poor glycemic control or small vessel diseases present (start at 26 weeks)
	If gestational diabetes order 2h 75 g OGTT
What percentage of gestational diabetes develops diabetes after pregnancy?	35%
When do you see caudal regression syndrome?	Seen with overt diabetes
When do you see strong association between congenital abnormalities and HbA1c?	>8.5 strongly associated
When do you deliver if there is gestational diabetes?	At 40th or 39 week if of poor glycemic control & if <4500 g, however if >4500 g do C-section (risk of shoulder dystocia)
What L/S ratio is considered normal?	>2.5
Why do you have to stop insulin infusion right after delivery?	Sudden drop of diabetogenic hormones right after delivery leaves insulin without opposing effect and hypoglycemia develops
What are the neonatal problems of gestational diabetes?	Hypoglycemia, hypocalcemia, hypomagnesemia, low surfactant (RDS), polycythemia and jaundice
What is the mechanism of hypocalcemia in neonates of diabetic mother?	PTH synthesis is impaired
What is gestational	A mild and self limited low platelet

thrombocytopenia?	during pregnancy
What is the diagnosis of severe pruritus of palms and soles and no rash in a pregnant woman of European heritage with very high bile acids?	Intrahepatic cholestasis of pregnancy; treat with Ursodeoxycholic acid + antihistamines + cholestyramine
What rare disease can mimic pre-eclampsia?	Acute fatty liver
How do you treat UTI in pregnancy?	Asymptomatic bacteriuria and cystitis treated with nitrofurantoin, Pyelonephritis is treated with cephalosporins or gentamicin, also add tocolysis
How do you perform 1st trimester induced abortion?	Medical up to 63 days after amenorrhea : mifepristone (progesterone) plus misoprostol (prostaglandin) D&C up to 13 weeks
How do you perform 2nd trimester induced abortion?	Dilatation and evacuation or partial birth
What percentage of threatened abortion loses the fetus?	50%
What is the next step if ultrasound is showing no conception in a suspected incomplete abortion?	Follow with weekly hCG until it is negative
What is the diagnosis of unilateral pelvic pain, vaginal bleeding and amenorrhea?	

Ectopic pregnancy

What is the diagnosis of unilateral pelvic pain, vaginal bleeding, amenorrhea, hypotension & abdominal rigidity and guarding?	Ruptured ectopic pregnancy
What is the most common risk factor for ectopic pregnancy?	Pelvic inflammatory disease
How much the risk of ectopic pregnancy is increased by having a positive history of ectopic pregnancy?	From 1% goes to 15%
What is the value of hCG in ectopic pregnancy?	At 5 weeks of gestation must be >1500 (vaginal ultrasound) and at 6 weeks must be >6500 (abdominal ultrasound)
Can lack of adnexal mass rule out ectopic pregnancy?	No
What is the next step in suspected ectopic pregnancy if hCG is <1500?	Repeat hCG and ultrasound until >1500
How do you manage ectopic pregnancy?	Immediate surgery (salpingotomy)
How do you manage unruptured ectopic pregnancy?	Methotrexate and laparoscopy
When do you give methotrexate in ectopic pregnancy?	Mass is >3.5 cm, absence of fetal heart motion, hCG < 6000 and no history of folate supplementation

USMLE STEP 3 IN ONE WEEK

What is the one thing you have to do before cerclage?

Rule out chorioamnionitis

What are the risk factors for cervical insufficiency?

2nd trimester abortion, laceration of cervix, conization, DES use

What is the indication of cerclage?

Any patient with 3 or more unexplained 2nd trimester fetal loss needs cerclage at 13-16 weeks

When do you remove cerclage?

36-37 weeks when L/S >2.5

Can you do cerclage if there is no dilatation?

Not indicated unless 3 or more 2nd trimester fetal loss is in the history

What is IUGR?

< 5-10 percentile or <2500 g but accurate early pregnancy dating is needed for diagnosis

What are the causes of symmetric IUGR?

Fetal causes: TORCH, aneuploidy, structural abnormalities e.g. NTD, congenital heart diseases

What are the causes of asymmetric IUGR?

Maternal or placental
Maternal: HTN, vasculitis, malnutrition, cigarette, alcohol, drugs
Placental: abruption, placenta previa, infarction, twin-twin transfusion

What are the risk factors for macrosomia?

Diabetes and gestational diabetes, increase weight gain, multiparity, prolonged gestation

When do you perform elective C-section for macrosomia?

If >5000 g in non-diabetics & >4500 in diabetics

What is Erb's palsy?	C5 and C6 paralysis seen more in macrosomy
When you do ultrasound, CVS, amniocentesis, fetoscopy, cord blood sampling & cerclage?	Ultrasound: 10-13 weeks CVS: 12-14 Amniocentesis: 15 fetoscopy & cord blood sampling >20 cerclage: 13-24
How do you diagnose premature rupture of membrane?	Speculum examination shows clear fluid nitrazine test is positive ferning pattern positive ultrasound shows oligohydramnios
What are the signs of chorioamnionitis?	Fever, tenderness, confirmed premature rupture of membrane, absence of UTI or upper respiratory infection
How do you manage chorioamnionitis?	<24 weeks needs only bed rest 24-33 weeks: ampicillin + erythromycin + fluid + betamethasone 34 weeks and higher : delivery Cervical culture before antibiotics
What criteria needed for labor?	Every 2-3 min for 45-60 seconds and 50 mmHg contraction
When do you interfere with the second stage of labor?	When do you interfere with the second stage of labor? Add 1h for epidural
How do you manage prolonged stage II of labor?	If head is engaged forceps delivery and if not C-section

What are the causes of prolonged stage II of labor?	PPP: pelvis, power, passenger (fetus)
What are the phases of stage I labor?	Latent & active (when dilatation accelerates), latent is <14h or 20h depending on parity; active phase needs at least 1.2-1.5 cm/h depending on parity
What is the management for prolonged stage I labor?	Bed rest and sedation
What is the management for prolonged stage II labor?	If adequate contraction do C-section ; if hypotonic induce with oxytocin if hypertonic use morphine
How do you manage cord prolapse?	Knee chest position, terbutaline, emergency C-section
What is considered reassuring during fetal heart rate tracing?	Beat to beat variability & the heart rate is 120-160 acceleration is present and there is no deceleration
What is non-assuring fetal heart rate monitoring?	Brady or tachycardia: mostly drugs like beta agonists/antagonists can cause that deceleration (early or late), no acceleration, no beat to beat variability
What is the mechanism of early deceleration?	Fetal head compression
What is the mechanism of variable deceleration?	Cord compression and acidosis
What is the mechanism of late deceleration?	Uteroplacental insufficiency

What are the steps in the management of non-assuring FHR tracing?	Stop medication, high flow oxygen, lie on left side, IV fluid, vaginal exam to rule out cord prolapse, scalp stimulation to see acceleration, if none is helping delivery is the management
Can you use forceps if the orientation of the head is not clear?	No
What are the contraindications to forceps or vaccum?	No full dilatation, no ROM (rupture of membrane), no engagement of the presenting part, cephalopelvic disproportion, head orientation isn't clear
What are the indications of forceps or vaccum?	Prolonged 2nd stage of labor, non-reassuring fetal heart monitoring, mother can't or shouldn't push
What are the risks of C-section?	Bleeding, infection, visceral injury, DVT
When can you do external cephalic version?	Around 37th week if the lie is transverse or breech
What are the indications of C-section?	Cephalopelvic disproportion, transverse lie or breach, placenta previa, HIV, HSV, non-reassuring electronic fetal monitoring, history of classic C-section
What is the success rate with vaginal birth after C-section?	80%
What are the 6 causes of postpartum hemorrhage?	Atony: massage, oxytocin, methlyergonovine Retained placenta

	Laceration Uterine inversion DIC: caused by missed abortion, abruption, amniotic fluid embolism, severe toxemia Urinary retention
What is the best emergency contraception?	Copper IUD has 99% success rate and can be given up to five days after the incident
How do you manage postpartum contraception?	Breastfeeding is good for 12 weeks but can't be trusted; progestin can be started right after delivery ; combined oral contraceptives can start 3 weeks after delivery, IUD and diaphragm after 6 weeks postpartum
What are the differentials of postpartum fever?	0 day: atelectasis 1st day: UTI 2-3 days after: endometritis 4-5 days after: wound infection 5-6 days after: thrombophlebitis 7-21 days after: mastitis
Is it necessary to order CXR for suspicious atelectasis?	Not necessary
What is the risk of appendicitis to pregnant women?	2nd trimester premature birth, 3rd trimester rupture and peritonitis
How do you treat endometritis?	Gentamicin + clindamycin
What is the most common cause of nipple discharge?	Intraductal papilloma which can be bloody; discharge can be galactorrhea so rule out the common causes of that
Can you use cytology for ductal discharge to rule out malignancy?	No

USMLE STEP 3 IN ONE WEEK

What is the definite diagnosis of intraductal papilloma?	Duct excision unless it is bilateral or milky discharge is present
What is fibrocystic disease of the breast?	Bilateral painful cysts, pain changes during menstruation
How do you treat fibrocystic disease?	Oral contraceptives
What are different methods of breast biopsy?	Fine needle aspiration, core needle biopsy, open biopsy; open biopsy is used if bloody discharge or clinically is inflammatory carcinoma
How do you approach breast diseases?	If a cyst is felt during physical examination, do ultrasound and if there is a cyst do FNA if there is a mass and she is <40 do biopsy
How do you treat DCIS?	Lumpectomy, radiation and tamoxifen
What is the treatment of LCIS?	Only tamoxifen
What are the main forms of breast carcinoma?	Invasive ductal is 85 % of all cases, invasive lobular is 10%, inflammatory and Paget's disease of the breast
What are the risk factors for breast carcinoma?	>50, positive FH, positive history of breast carcinoma, 1st child after 30 or nulliparity, radiation or hormonal therapy, obesity, higher socioeconomic status, benign breast diseases
When is BRCA testing indicated?	Breast or ovary carcinoma in the same patient, family history of male breast carcinoma, early onset family history, Aschkenazi Jewish
When is chemotherapy the main treatment for breast	If metastasis seen, if >5 cm, if inflammatory carcinoma seen

carcinoma?

Can breast conserving surgery be used if there is history of radiation?	No
When do you use adjuvant hormonal therapy?	If the tumor is positive for hormone receptor
What is the result of 5 years treatment with tamoxifen?	50% decrease in recurrence 25% decrease in mortality
What are the aromatase inhibitors?	Anastrazole, letrozole, exemestane they cause no menopausal symptoms but do cause osteoporosis
What are the alternatives to tamoxifen?	Aromatase inhibitors, ovarian ablation, HGRH analogue (goserelin)
What are the disadvantages of tamoxifen?	Endometrial carcinoma, menopausal symptoms get worse
What are the advantages of tamoxifen?	Decrease chance of contralateral breast carcinoma, increase bone density and decrease bone fractures, decrease cardiovascular mortality and decrease cholesterol
When do you add chemotherapy?	When tumor >1 cm or positive node is found
When do you use trastuzumab?	HER 2/neu positive and there is metastasis
What is the difference between trastuzumab anthrycyline cardiotoxicity?	Trastuzumab is reversible
How do you choose chemotherapy in pre and post-	If hormone receptor negative use chemotherapy alone, if hormone

menopausal women with breast carcinoma?	receptor positive add tamoxifen if premenopausal and if postmenopausal add aromatase inhibitors
What are the differentials for uterus enlargement?	Leiomyoma : asymmetric nontender adenomyosis: symmetric tender pregnancy
What race has very high chance of leiomyoma?	Black race has five times more, growth increases in pregnancy and decreases after menopause
What is the parasitic leiomyoma?	Subserosal leiomyoma gets its blood supply from omentum or intestinal mesentery
How do you treat leiomyoma?	If post fertility you can do hysterectomy, serial examination and observation, goserelin for 3-6 months can reduce the size for surgery, myomectomy (other pregnancies will be C-section , embolization of vessels)
What is the treatment for adenomyosis?	IUD with levonorgesterol, if post fertility do hysterectomy
What is the most important risk factor for endometrial carcinoma?	Unopposed estrogen effect: chronic form is seen in PCOS and chronic anovulation, nulliparity, early menarche and late menopause
How do you diagnose endometrial carcinoma?	Pelvic exam and biopsy: atrophy needs hormone replacement, adenocarcinoma needs surgery and staging plus radiotherapy or chemotherapy hysteroscopy: rule out polyps as source

of bleeding   Ultrasound: measure endometrial thickness if <5 mm in postmenopausal women is normal

What kind of surgery is done for adenocarcinoma of uterus?	THA + BSO + pelvic and paraaortic lymphadenectomy + peritoneal washing
When do you give chemotherapy for uterine adenocarcinoma?	If it is metastatic
When do you use radiation?	Node involvement, >50% myometrial invasion, positive surgical margin, poorly differentiated
What are the seven causes of ovarian enlargement?	Physiologic cyst Complex cyst PCOS Hyperthecosis Luteoma of pregnancy Theca lutein cyst Neoplasm
How do you manage ovarian physiologic cyst?	They are asymptomatic unless torsion happens; treat with follow up after 6-8 weeks, most of them disappear, prevent by oral contraceptive, if >7 cm or persistent after oral contraceptives remove laparoscopically
What is the management of hyperthecosis?	Oral contraceptive suppresses androgen by LH stimulation
How do you workup an ovarian mass?	hCG, ultrasound, if >7 cm laparoscopy or laparotomy
Which side is more common to have ovarian torsion?	Right

How do you treat ovarian torsion?	laparoscopic removal unless there is necrosis which needs oophorectomy; follow up in 4 weeks
What is the next step in ovarian enlargement in prepubertal or postmenopausal women?	Rule out neoplasm
What are the risk factors for ovarian carcinoma?	BRCA, family history, high number of ovulation, talc powder, infertility
What are the protective factors against ovarian tumors?	Decrease ovulation: oral contraceptives, anovulation, breast feeding, short reproductive life
How do you evaluate a patient suspected of ovarian neoplasm?	Do CT if no ascites do laparoscopic oophorectomy; if ascites present do surgical staging and oophorectomy
What are the 5 forms of ovarian cancer and tumor markers for each of them?	Dysgerminoma (children): AFP, LDH, hCG epithelial tumors: CEA and CA 125 granulosa-theca tumor: estrogen gastric cancer metastasis: mucin producing tumor
How do you manage ovarian tumors?	Ultrasound or CT (pot menopausal) laparoscopic biopsy tumor markers cystectomy for benign cyst TAH + BSO + chemotherapy in postmenopausal; if premenopausal salpingo-oophorectomy is done
Which human papilloma viruses have malignant potential?	16, 18, 31, 33, 35

Which HPV viruses are causing condyloma acuminate?	6, 11
How do you manage ASCUS (atypia of squamous cells of undetermined significance)?	HPV DNA testing or repeat Pap if any of these two positive colposcopy and biopsy is done
What is the next step for LSIL or low grade squamous intraepithelial lesion (CIN I)?	Observe and follow up : repeat Pap smear and colposcopy
What is the next step for HSIL (CIS, CIN 2 or 3)? **How do you manage cervical cancer?**	Ablation or excision Simple of modified radical hysterectomy
What is the workup plan in metastatic cervical tumor?	Pelvic exam, CXR, IVP, cystoscopy, sigmoidoscopy, no need for CT/MRI for staging
What do you add radiotherapy and chemotherapy?	If tumor is >4 cm, if adenopathy is present, positive margins, local recurrence, if poorly differentiated
What is Gardasil?	6,11, 16 & 18 strains of HPV virus vaccine; it is not recommended for pregnancy, lactating women, immunocompromised
What are the causes for pelvic pain?	cervicitis, acute salpingooophoritis, chronic PID, tubo-ovarian abscess
How do you workup for pelvic pain?	Pelvic exam, cervical culture, ESR, WBC, ultrasound
How do you treat cervicitis?	Azithromycin + cefixime
What is the treatment for	Outpatient: ofloxacin + metronidazole

acute salpingo-oophoritis?	inpatient: gentamicin + clindamycin/doxycycline + cefoxitin/cefotetan
What are the main signs and risk factors of PID?	FAD: fever, abdominal pain and discharge are seen in pelvic inflammatory disease Risk factors: <35, multiple partners, lack of barrier, douching, PMH of PID
What is the treatment for chronic pelvic inflammatory diseases?	Adhesion lysis, severe cases need TAH + BSO
What is pelvic inflammatory disease?	Infection above cervix; the chronic form has infertility+ dyspareunia, bilateral hydrosalpinx
How do you treat PID?	Doxycycline and ceftriaxone/cefotaxime Or clindamycin and gentamicin
What is the diagnosis of a patient with sever pelvic pain, very high ESR, severe leukocytosis, fever, vomiting, tachycardia, pus on culdocentesis, unilateral mass on ultrasound and anaerobes growth on blood culture?	Tubo-ovarian abscess Treatment: admit, clindamycin + gentamicin IV, if no response within 72h surgery is performed
When do you admit PID?	Nulligravida, adolescence, IUD, fever, abscess, outpatient failed before
What is dysmenorrhea?	Crampy pain, nausea, vomiting, diarrhea because of PGF2
What are different types of dysmenorrhea?	Primary dysmenorrhea is within 2-5 years of first menstruation, secondary is later in life and the causes are: endometriosis, adenomyosis, leiomyoma

How do you treat dysmenorrhea?	1st line: NSAIDS for 2-4 months; 2nd line: oral contraceptives
What is the most common location for endometriosis?	Ovary shows chocolate cysts Douglas pouch: uteroscacral ligament shows nodularity; uterus is retroverted
What is the relationship between endometriosis and CA 125?	Can be elevated
How do you diagnose endometriosis?	Laparoscopy
How do you treat endometriosis?	Oral contraceptive or continuous progesterone testosterone derivatives (danazol) or leuprolide (GnRH analogue), laparoscopic lysis, TAH & BSO
What are the causes of premenarchal bleeding?	Foreign body, trauma, abuse, tumors of ovaries or pituitary, precocious puberty, sarcoma botryoides
What is considered primary amenorrhea?	At 14 if no secondary sexual characteristics and at 16 is they are present
What is the workup for primary amenorrhea?	hCG, ultrasound, HSPG, karyotyping, testosterone, FSH
What is considered secondary amenorrhea?	if regular menses 3 months of no menses otherwise 6 months of no menses
How do you treat androgen	estrogen replacement, removal of

insensitivity?	abdominal testes before 20 years of age
What is Kallman's syndrome?	anosmia + hypopituitarism, CT head to rule out tumors; treat with estrogen and progesterone replacement
What is the relationship between TRH and prolactin?	TRH is the releasing hormone for TSH and prolactin
What is the workup for secondary amenorrhea?	hCG, TSH, prolactin, progesterone challenge test & estrogen challenge test
What is the importance of a positive progesterone challenge test?	It means there is withdrawal bleeding i.e. no ovulation; treat with clomiphene and cyclic progesterone to counter unopposed estrogen
What if the next step is there is negative progesterone challenge test?	If progesterone challenge test is negative do HSPG which can show outflow obstruction or Asherman syndrome; if the test is positive and FSH is high it is ovarian failure and if it is low, it is hypopituitarism
What is premenstrual dysphoric disorder?	Daily functioning is disturbed treat with SSRI, B6 and diuretics
What is the hirsutism workup?	Testosterone, DHEAS, LH/FSH, 17 hydroxyprogesterone
What is the diagnosis amenorrhea + unpredictable bleeding?	Anovulation
What are the causes of anovulation?	PCOS, medication, prolactin, hypothyroidism, pituitary adenoma
What is the LH/FSH ratio in PCOS?	Elevated : 3 to 1 as opposed to normal value (1.5:1)

USMLE STEP 3 IN ONE WEEK

How do you manage PCOS?	Oral contraceptives, spironolactone, clomiphene, statins, metformin
What hormones are responsible for adrenal and ovarian virilization?	DHEAS in adrenal and testosterone in ovary
What is the diagnosis if during 2nd or 3rd decade there is gradual hirsutism and negative ovulation and no virilization?	Measure 17 hydroxyprogesterone and if positive 21 hydroxylase deficiency is the diagnosis
How do you teat idiopathic hirsutism?	Spironolactone and topical eflorinthine
How do you diagnose menopause?	Serial FSH and LH with 3 months of amenorrhea
What do you call menopause before 30 years?	Premature ovarian failure
What is menopause between 30 to 40 years of age?	Premature menopause
What percentage of menopause women has hot flashes?	75%
Wehat maedication helps with sleep problems and vasomotor signs in post menopausal women?	venlafaxine
What are the risk factors for osteoporosis?	steroids, thin, smoker, low calcium, white, sedentary lifestyle, history of low impact fracture, malabsorption
When do you need to do bone densitometry?	Over 65 if there is no risk factors otherwise at 58
How do you interpret T score	T score is the standard deviation from

in DEXA scan?	the mean; >2.5 is osteoporosis; 1.0-2.5 is osteopenic
How do you check for bone breakdown?	24h Urine NTX (N-telopeptide), hydroxyproline
What is the treatment of osteoporosis?	1st line: bisphosphonates or SERM 2nd line: calcitonin and fluoride
Can we use estrogen for treating osteoporosis?	Never
What are the indications of hormone replacement therapy?	Vasomotor signs, urinary complaints and dyspareunia
What are the benefits of HRT?	Decrease osteoporotic fractures, decrease colorectal cancer
What are the risks of HRT?	DVT, heart attack, breast cancer (if >4 years use)
What are the advantages of low dose oral contraceptive pills?	No increased risk of cancer, heart diseases, thromboembolism
What is the mechanism of PCOS?	Insulin resistance causing high insulin which causes high androgen production & PCOS
What is the absolute contraindication for oral contraceptives?	Pregnancy, acute liver disease, DVT, CVA, SLE, hormone dependent breast cancer, smoker over 35, uncontrolled HTN or 160/100, migraine with aura, thrombophilia, diabetes with vascular diseases
What are the relative	Diabetes, HTN, migraine,

contraindications for oral contraceptives?	hyperlipidemia, depression
What are the benefits of oral contraceptives?	Decrease ovarian & endometrial cancer, decrease dysmenorrhea, DUB (dysfunctional uterine bleeding), ectopic pregnancy
What are the absolute contraindications of IUD?	Pregnancy, pelvic malignancy, salpingitis
What are the relative contraindications of IUD?	Nulliparity, history of ectopic pregnancy, abnormal Pap smear, abnormal uterine shape, immune suppression
What are the first and second steps in infertility workup?	1st: semen analysis and if abnormal repeat after 4-6 weeks; 2nd is testing ovulation and tube patency
What is the normal semen analysis?	>20 million, >50% motile, >50% normal morphology, > 2 ml volume, pH between 7.2-7.8
What is the mechanism of estrogen in treating DUB?	Dysfunctional uterine bleeding is stopped by estrogen since it helps with hemostasis
How do you do anovulation workup?	BBT (basal body temperature), progesterone level, endometrial biopsy
What is the workup for tube abnormalities?	HSPG, laparoscopy, Chlamydia serology (IgG) and if negative infection as a cause is ruled out
What percentage of unexplained infertilities gets pregnant is 3 years?	60%
What is the success rate of	55%

four cycles of IVF?

What cells are involved in gestational trophoblastic disease?	Both syncitiotrophoblasts and cytotrophoblasts
Which race has the highest rate for GTD?	Taiwan and Philippines
What is the diagnosis of a pregnant woman with bleeding before 16th week and has passed vesicles, no FHR, uterus is bigger than expected, bilateral cystic enlargement of ovaries also seen?	GTD (mole): 1. Complete (empty egg), has 20% chance of malignancy, 46XX and no fetus 2. Incomplete has normal egg with dead fetus (69 XXY), 10% chance of malignancy 3. Choriocarcinoma: nonmetastatic has 100 % cure rate; metastatic without brain or liver has 95% and if brain or liver involved 65% are cured
Why do we give oral contraceptives in mole?	To ensure there is no pregnancy is occurred and the results of hCG is not mixed. hCG is needed for following up mole.

Psychiatry, Ethics & Intoxications

What are positive symptoms?	Agitation, delusion, hallucination, disorganized speech or behavior
What are negative symptoms?	Apathy, social withdrawal, anhedonia, flattened affect, poverty of thought
What atipsychotics are most effective for negative symptoms?	CROZAC: clozapine (agranulocytosis)) , risperidone, olanzapine, ziprasidone, quetiapine
What are the schizophrenia, schizophreniform and brief psychotic disorders?	>6 months is schizophrenia, 1-6 months is schizophreniform, <1 month is brief psychotic disorders
What are the differentials for non-bizarre delusions for a long time?	Schizotypal personality disorder or delusional disorders
What is the next step if antipsychotics don't work for schizophrenia?	Psychotherapy
What is the workup for schizophrenia?	Drug screening, check for seizure signs or symptoms which can show temporal lobe epilepsy, watch for suicidal ideations
What is the greatest risk factor for schizophrenia?	Schizophreniform disorder (2/3 develop schizophrenia)
Who has better prognosis of schizophrenia?	Girls and paranoid form

What are the signs of poor prognosis in schizophrenia?	Early onset, negative symptoms, family history, disorganized or deficit type, poor premorbid functioning
How do you manage schizophrenia?	If paranoid or bizarre admit, benzodiazepines used first and then antipsychotics (for 6 months if another episode is seen use them for longer), long term psychotherapy
What are the main indications of antipsychotics?	1. Schizophrenia and other psychotic disorders, Sedation when benzodiazepines are contraindicated 2. Movement disorders e.g. Huntington's disease & Tourette
What are the conventional antipsychotics?	High potency: haloperidol, fluphenazine; these are less sedating but has more EPS syndromes Low potency: thioridazine (long QT syndrome), chlorpromazine; these are less EPS but more sedation and anticholinergic
What is the next step if a patient is taking thioridazine comes with chest pain?	EKG to rule out arrhythmia
What is the most common reason for lack of compliance in using antipsychotics?	Male: impotence and problem with ejaculation Female: hyperprolactinemia and weight gain
What antipsychotic is	Thioridazine

causing retinal pigmentation?	
What is used in schizophrenia if sedation is required for insomnia?	Olanzapine, quetiapine, ziprasidone, aripiprazole
What is used if too much of sedation & sleepiness is seen?	Risperidone
What are the EPS movement disorders?	Parkinsonism: decrease the dose, give benztropine Akathesia: a motor restlessness, give beta blocker or benzodiazepines Acute dystonia: benztropine can help tardive dyskinesia : can happen even after stopping the medication NMS: admit ICU; fever, high CK and WBC
What is the most effective antipsychotic?	Clozapine but its dangerous side effects (seizure & agranulocytosis) makes it 2nd line
How do you monitor patient with clozapine?	Weekly blood check for 6 months and then bimonthly and finally monthly
What are the main causes of catatonia (a state of apparent unresponsiveness?	Psychotic dis. Mood disorder with psychotic features, autism spectrum disorders and medical conditions
What are the main features of anxiety disorders?	No identifiable cause while disturbing daily life
How do you diagnose generalized anxiety disorders?	At least 3 of MERISCH Muscle tension, easy fatigability, restlessness, sleep problems, concentration affected and hypervigilance
What are the causes of	Hyperthyroidism, pheochromocytoma,

anxiety?	heart failure, COPD, asthma, arrhythmia, hypercortisolism, stimulant drugs and withdrawal from alcohol or sedatives
How do you treat adjustment disorders?	Counselling
How do you manage panic disorders?	CBT (cognitive behavior therapy), SSRI, benzodiazepines, TCA, MAO
What is the treatment for phobia?	Exposure, benzodiazepines, beta blockers
What are the complications of insight in OCD?	Depression and drug abuse
What is the treatment of OCD?	SSRI & behavior therapy
How long is acute stress disorder?	<1 month duration
What is the duration of PTSD?	>1 month duration of avoidance, increased arousal & flash backs
How do you treat PTSD?	For acute cases benzodiazepines, SSRI for long term, group therapy right after the event helps
What is GAD?	>6 months and no single event is responsible, they have multiple life circumstances
How do you treat GAD?	Treatment: psychotherapy, benzodiazepines, SSRI, venlafaxine (SNRI), buspirone
What is the order of duration of action of	Alprazolam<lorazepam<diazepam

benzodiazepines used frequently?	
What is the main advantage of buspirone?	Less sedative, best for driving or working with machinery, no withdrawal
What do you have to rule out to diagnose major depressive disorders?	More than 2 weeks of anhedonia is needed but you should rule out thyroid disorders, medications (beta blockers, antipsychotics), substance abuse and Parkinson's disease
What is dysthymia?	Mild depression for >2 years; long term insight oriented psychotherapy is used; 2nd line is SSRI
How do you treat seasonal affective disorders?	Phototherapy or sleep deprivation
How do you diagnose bipolar disorders?	At least one week of mania/depression/mixed symptoms is needed for the diagnosis
What is the treatment of bipolar disorders?	Admit, risperidone for acute mania, Li, intramuscular depot of phenothiazines if noncompliant
When do you use antidepressants in bipolar disorders?	Use them only with lithium if recurrent depression is seen, they can cause rapid cycling bipolar disorders
What is rapid cycling bipolar disorders?	If >4 episodes in one year
How do you prevent rapid cycling bipolar disorders?	Gradually stop benzodiazepines, caffeine, alcohol, stimulants & antidepressants

What is the relationship between hypothyroidism and rapid cycling bipolar disorders?	Cause and effect
What drugs do decrease suicide in bipolar disorders?	Li but don't use it in pregnancy
How do you treat bipolar disorders in pregnancy? What is cyclothymia and its treatment?	ECT, lamotrigine is 2nd line >2 years of hypomania and depressed mood; treat with psychotherapy ; if function is impaired divalproex is used
What is the main difference between grief and depression?	Grief has normal level of functioning after 2 months and doesn't last more than a year, it has no feeling of guilt or shame
If a patient has both psychotic and mood symptoms which one do you treat first?	Treat psychotic symptoms first
When do you give SSRI in grief?	If > 6 months and symptoms are like depression Note : Auditory hallucinations are common in grief
How do you treat postpartum depression?	Antidepressants, if postpartum blue then no need to treat, of postpartum psychosis use antipsychotics & antidepressants unless breast feeding (use ECT)
What are the risk factors for suicide?	History of attempts or threats , male , family history , >65 , schizophrenia , borderline or antisocial personality disorder, socially isolated , loss of job,

	chronic illnesses
What is suicide emergency assessment?	Take all threats seriously, detain and hospitalize (usually for a couple of weeks) , never transport the patient without medical personnel, don't identify with the patient, treat with SSRI & antipsychotics and if acute use ECT
What are the indications of ECT?	Good response in the past, contraindication to medications, failure of medications
What are ECT complications?	Headache, transient memory loss, increased ICP transiently , caution in space occupying lesions
How do you treat depression?	6 months unless multiple episodes which needs longer treatment SSRI are first line but if it doesn't show any effect in 8 weeks change them. Use bupropion if weight gain or sexual side effects are the problems; mirtazapine is used for poor sleep/appetite/ weight loss; if severe insomnia use trazodone
Can you use SSRI or TCA in pregnancy?	Safe except for paroxetine
What are the indications of SSRI?	MDD, anxiety disorders (GAD , OCD, panic disorders, social phobia), bipolar, bulimic
For how long do you treat MDD?	6-12 months after symptom free
What are the most important side effects of trazodone?	Priapism
What is the treatment of depression + agitation?	Doxepin or trazodone

What antidepressant can be used for chronic pain?	Amitriptyline
What medications are not used in depression and seizure?	Bupropion and TCA
What is the diagnosis of a drug overdosed patient with hypotension, tachycardia and mydriasis?	TCA overdose; manage with EKG and sodium bicarbonate, charcoal within first 2h unless ileus is present
When do you use divalproex?	When lithium isn't effective and in rapid cycling bipolar disorders
What are the effects of lithium on thyroid gland?	Hypo and hyperthyroidism, goiter, autoimmune thyroiditis
What medications do have interaction with lithium?	ACEI, ARB, NSAIDS, SSRI, diuretics and antiepileptics
When do you use carbamazepine for bipolar disorders?	2nd line of therapy for bipolar disorders; sedation and agranulocytosis are the side effects
What are the features of Li toxicity?	Tremor, renal failure, seizure, increased DTR, nausea and vomiting
What are the major features of narcolepsy?	Cataplexy, low hypocretin 1, low REM latency
How do you treat narcolepsy?	Modafinil For catalepsy use Sodium oxybate or venlafaxine
What are the causes of neuroleptic malignant syndrome?	This is a dopamine blockade syndrome (very high fever, tachycardia, rigidity, loss of consciousness, autonomic dysfunction) which is seen in Parkinson's diseases who stopped levodopa, and patients who recently started haloperidol
How do you treat NMS?	Treat with bromocriptine, dantrolene

	and diazepam
What is serotonin syndrome?	Similar to NMS and usually happens after the use of SSRI + MAO or antimigraines (-triptans) but treatment is cyproheptadine and benzodiazepines
What is the first thing to consider when prescribing SSRI?	Suicidal ideation can increase in the first 2 weeks of use; treat with stopping the medication and consider ECT
What do you need for diagnosing somatization disorder?	4211: 4 pain; 2 GI; one sexual and one pseudoneurologic
What is the main feature of conversion disorder?	No insight
How do you diagnose hypochondriasis?	>6 months despite negative tests and despite physician assurance
What is the main feature of malingering?	Reward and secondary gain
What percentage of anorexia nervosa has purging symptoms?	50%
What causes cardiomyopathy in bulimic patients?	IPECAC overuse
How do you treat anorexia nervosa or bulimia?	Admit, IV fluid, correct electrolytes, olanzapine helps with weight, SSRI prevent relapse, behavior psychotherapy
How do you treat body dysmorphic disorders?	High dose SSRI

USMLE STEP 3 IN ONE WEEK

What are impulse control disorders?	Intermittent explosive disorders Kleptomania Pyromania (starts a fight with no 2° gain) Pathologic gambling
What is number one cause of injury to women in the US?	Physical abuse by spouse; reporting is not indicated but provide shelter & counseling information
What are the risk factors for physical abuse in women?	Pregnant, dependent personality, young age marriage, history of violent home for victim when show grows up; drugs & alcohol
Child abuse must be less than what age that must be reported?	Less than 18 years of age must be reported
Is female circumcision a form of abuse?	Yes
What are the personality disorders?	Cluster A : weird (schizoid, schizotypal, paranoid) Cluster B: wild (histrionic, antisocial, narcissistic, borderline) Cluster C: worried (OCPD, dependent, avoidant)
What personality disorder is associated with hypochondriasis?	Borderline, histrionic, dependent
In what personality disorder mutilation and self- aggression is seen?	Passive aggressive
Who is a heavy drinker?	Male: >7 per week

USMLE STEP 3 IN ONE WEEK

What is moderate drinking?	Female: >14/week Male 2 per day and female 1 per day is moderate alcohol which has positive effects on hear and blood pressure
How do you manage alcohol withdrawal?	If acute inpatient: thiamine, Mg, B12, folate, chlordiazepoxide unless liver disease then give lorazepam or oxazepam; if seizure give diazepam If acute outpatient: prevent, sedate and transfer If chronic: group therapy and drug therapy (only with group therapy use drugs like acamprosate/naloxone)
What is the most effective management of alcohol abuse and prevention of relapse?	AA (Alcoholics Anonymous)
What are the clinical features of minor alcohol withdrawal syndrome?	Onset after last drink is 6h , symptoms are insomnia, diaphoresis, palpitation, headache, tremulousness; treat with benzodiazepines
What kind of hallucination is seen in alcoholics?	12-24h after last drink usually visual hallucination is seen though it maybe tactile or auditory
When do you see withdrawal seizure in alcoholics?	After 2 days of last drink tonic-clonic seizure is seen; if repeats do CT
When do you see delirium tremens?	2-4 days after the last drink fever, tachycardia, tremor, diaphoresis, HTN, agitation & hallucination
When do you give mechanical ventilation in alcoholics?	If there is severe alcohol intoxication

How do you treat amphetamine or cocaine withdrawal?	Withdrawal : antidepressants ; intoxication; antipsychotics
What are the main features of cannabis intoxication?	Dry mouth, increased appetite, tachycardia, red eyes, social withdrawal
How do you treat barbiturate or benzodiazepine withdrawal?	Short acting barbiturates
How do you treat opiated withdrawal and intoxication?	Methadone and clonidine for withdrawal; naloxone for intoxication
How do you treat PCP/LSD/inhalants intoxication?	Antipsychotics
What is the main alpha 1 blockade side effect?	Impaired ejaculation
What is the main sexual side effect of SSRI?	Inhibits orgasm (good for treating premature ejaculation)
What is the main sexual side effect of dopamine?	Increased erection and libido
What are the side effects of neuroleptics and beta blockers?	Erectile dysfunction
What is considered paraphilia?	>6 months and affects level of functioning

USMLE STEP 3 IN ONE WEEK

What is frotteurism?	Touching and robbing
What is the 1st step in the management of drug overdose if ABC of CPR is alright?	Thiamine, dextrose, naloxone
Do we use IPECAC in children?	Never
Is charcoal a good choice for intoxication?	No
What is the antidote for methemoglobinemia?	Methylene blue
What is the antidote for NMS?	Bromocriptine and dantrolene
When do you give N acetylecysteine?	It is safe to use in all with possible acetaminophen toxicity
When it is late to stop acetaminophen toxicity on liver?	After 24h
What is the toxic and lethal dose of acetaminophen?	10g is toxic and 15 g is lethal
What are the main features of aspirin toxicity?	Tinnitus, ARDS, metabolic acidosis and fever (uncoupling oxidative phosphorylation), respiratory alkalosis, renal failure, high PT & INR, coma, seizure
For what intoxications do you add 3 ampules of bicarbonate to D5W?	TCA, aspirin, phenobarbital, chlorpropamide

What are the AAA levels used in all overdose cases?	Alcohol, aspirin, acetaminophen
How dangerous is benzodiazepine overdose?	Not fatal; supportive treatment is enough; don't give flumazenil because it can cause withdrawal & seizure if there is dependency to benzodiazepine; note that this seizure doesn't respond to benzodiazepines
What percentage of carbon monoxide intoxication in fire dies?	60%
What are the main features of digoxin toxicity?	GI upset, yellow halo, arrhythmia, encephalopathy, heperkalemia (Na/K pump isn't working well)
What acid base disorder is common between methanol and ethylene glycol intoxications?	Increased AG metabolic acidosis
What renal & electrolyte disorders do you see with ethylene glycol intoxication?	kidney stones and failure, hypocalcemia because of oxalate
What is the main feature of methemoglobinemia?	Normal PO2 and dark color of blood
What causes methemoglobinemia?	Caused by dapsone, nitrates, local anesthetics with –caine suffix, oxidants; treatment is 100% O2 and methylene blue
Does anyone die from opiate withdrawal or	No mortality from withdrawal but intoxication is treated with naloxone

USMLE STEP 3 IN ONE WEEK

intoxication?

What is the diagnosis of acute abdomen, no tenderness, but pain and rigidity present?	If hypocalcemia is present think of black widow spider; treat with Ca and antivenin
How do you diagnose brown recluse spider bite?	Local necrosis, bullae, dark lesion
How do you treat brown recluse spider bite?	Debridement and maybe steroids and dapsone
What is the respiratory management of a patient saved from fire?	100% O2 then intubate if hoarseness, wheeze, stridor, burns inside nose and mouth
How do you calculate fluid loss in burn?	4 ml/ kg / percentage of body burnt
What is the EKG sign of hypothermia?	J waves of Osborne which is similar to ST elevation
What is the diagnosis of fixed midsize pupils in a red eye?	Acute glaucoma is an emergency and should be treated with pilocarpine or timolol
How do you treat retinal detachment?	Tilt the head back, reattach by surgery/ cryo / injection of gas in the eye, put a band around the eye to get sclera close to retina
What are the differentials for red eye syndrome?	Conjunctivitis, uveitis, corneal abrasion & glaucoma
Which herbal supplements do cause bleeding?	Black cohesh, Ginkgo biloba, Ginseng, Saw palmetto
What are the main adverse effects of licorice?	HTN and hypokalemia
What is the purpose of	Insomnia but it is hepatotoxic and

using kava and what are its adverse effects?	causes somnolence
What is the importance of autonomy?	Respecting autonomy is more important than beneficence. Anybody with capacity can refuse any form of treatment
What are the differences between capacity and competence?	Competence is determined by a judge and capacity by a doctor
When there is no need to consult psychiatrist?	In coma or if the patient is clearly competent
What is considered partial emancipation?	Reproductive health, sex, substance abuse
Is there any universal law in the US regarding abortion and partial emancipation?	No. Most states wouldn't consider under 18 to be emancipated when abortion is the problem
Can parents refuse lifesaving therapy for their children?	No. Children are the property of state.
What are the main parts of informed consent?	Benefits, risks & alternatives
Is consent over the phone valid?	Yes
Can pregnant women refuse therapy?	Yes. Fetus is considered a part of her body
What are the exceptions to confidentiality?	Transmissible diseases e.g. HIV, psychiatric diseases with clear danger of injuring others
When is health care proxy valid?	Only if the patient has no capacity

What is very important in living will?	It must be clear
What is DNR?	No CPR but you do other tests and therapeutic measures
When do you need to contact ethics committee in hospital?	No clear wishes and no capacity, family members split or in disagreement about the nature of care
Can you provide pain medication to stop pain even if ends life?	Yes
When you don't have to provide care?	Brain death, futile treatment
How do you determine brain death?	1. Massive cortical destruction causing deep coma; EEG is flat 2. Lack of all brain stem reflexes 3. Medulla destruction with irreversible apnea 4. Rule out hypothermia/intoxication
What is impaired physician?	Must be reported if potential danger to medical care
Do you have to report elder abuse?	Can be reported against patient will
Can psychiatrists have sexual relationship with their patients?	Never, other specialties can stop seeing patient and then it is alright
Does the mother have always abortion right?	No rights during 3rd trimester

What are the contraindications of kidney transplantation?	Substance abuse, acute infection and HIV, malignancy, less than 18 and lack of capacity, certain kidney diseases, donor coercion, pregnancy

www.ingramcontent.com/pod-product-compliance
Lightning Source LLC
Chambersburg PA
CBHW052247220526
45471CB00001B/223